Hematology
Case Review

Hematology
Case Review

Donald C. Doll, MD

Professor Emeritus
Division of Hematology/Medical Oncology
Department of Internal Medicine
University of Missouri/Ellis Fischel Cancer Center
Columbia, Missouri

Radwan F. Khozouz, MD

Division of Hematology/Medical Oncology
Department of Internal Medicine
University of Missouri/Ellis Fischel Cancer Center
Columbia, Missouri

Wes Matthew Triplett, MD

Division of Hematology/Medical Oncology
Department of Internal Medicine
University of Missouri/Ellis Fischel Cancer Center
Columbia, Missouri

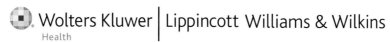
Wolters Kluwer | Lippincott Williams & Wilkins
Health

Philadelphia • Baltimore • New York • London
Buenos Aires • Hong Kong • Sydney • Tokyo

Senior Executive Editor: Jonathan W. Pine, Jr.
Senior Product Manager: Emilie Moyer
Production Product Manager: David Saltzberg
Manufacturing Manager: Beth Welsh
Marketing Manager: Stephanie Manzo
Art Director: Jennifer Clements
Senior Designer: Stephen Druding
Production Service: S4Carlisle

Printed in China

Library of Congress Cataloging-in-Publication Data

Doll, Donald C., author.
  Hematology case review / Donald C. Doll, Radwan F. Khozouz, Wes Matthew Triplett.—First edition.
    p. ; cm.
  Includes bibliographical references.
  ISBN 978-1-4511-9143-1
  I. Khozouz, Radwan F., 1980- author.   II. Triplett, Wes, Matthew, 1973- author.   III. Title.
  [DNLM: 1. Hematologic Diseases—diagnosis—Case Reports.   2. Hematologic Tests—Case Reports.
  WH 120]
  RC641.7.H35
  616.1'5—dc23

                                                                                    2013028399

Care has been taken to confirm the accuracy of the information presented and to describe generally accepted practices. However, the authors, editors, and publisher are not responsible for errors or omissions or for any consequences from application of the information in this book and make no warranty, expressed or implied, with respect to the currency, completeness, or accuracy of the contents of the publication. Application of the information in a particular situation remains the professional responsibility of the practitioner.

The authors, editors, and publisher have exerted every effort to ensure that drug selection and dosage set forth in this text are in accordance with current recommendations and practice at the time of publication. However, in view of ongoing research, changes in government regulations, and the constant flow of information relating to drug therapy and drug reactions, the reader is urged to check the package insert for each drug for any change in indications and dosage and for added warnings and precautions. This is particularly important when the recommended agent is a new or infrequently employed drug.

Some drugs and medical devices presented in the publication have Food and Drug Administration (FDA) clearance for limited use in restricted research settings. It is the responsibility of the health care provider to ascertain the FDA status of each drug or device planned for use in their clinical practice.

To purchase additional copies of this book, call our customer service department at (800) 638-3030 or fax orders to (301) 223-2320. International customers should call (301) 223-2300.

Visit Lippincott Williams & Wilkins on the Internet: at LWW.com. Lippincott Williams & Wilkins customer service representatives are available from 8:30 am to 6:00 pm, EST.

10 9 8 7 6 5 4 3 2 1

RRS1308

Dr. Triplett—for Aurora and Jackson; Dr. Khozouz—to Maria and Emma; Dr. Doll—to my beautiful wife, Christine, and my children, Christopher Joseph and Missy Angel.

Hematology is a fascinating adventure involving the study of blood cells. Interpretation of peripheral blood smears and bone marrow aspirates is an integral part of the science of hematology. For the past 40 years, one of the authors (DCD) has collected blood smears and bone marrow aspirates from patients encountered in his clinical practice. Images of blood specimens from these patients evaluated by the senior author form the basis of the case reports included in this book. Such cases vary from benign disorders, such as hereditary spherocytosis, to neoplastic disorders like acute leukemia. Both common and rare conditions are included, with the presenting symptoms, blood counts, and pertinent images, which are followed by questions and answers in a problem-based format. These cases have been used as a teaching tool for the past 15 years for medical students, medical residents, hematology-oncology fellows, and pathology residents. In addition, general internists, family practice physicians, and hospitalists may find this material useful in their daily encounters of patients with abnormal blood counts.

Donald C. Doll, MD
Radwan F. Khozouz, MD
Wes Matthew Triplett, MD
Christopher J. Doll, MPA

We would like to thank our administrative staff, Theresa Murphy, for her never-ending support, and Jonathan W. Pine, Jr, Emilie Moyer, Nicole Dernoski, and Jeff Gunning of Lippincott Williams and Wilkins for believing and supporting this project. In addition, we would like to thank all of the students, medical residents, hematopathologists, hematology-oncology fellows, and colleagues-especially William Caldwell, Michael Wang, Michael Perry, Joe Lezama, and Carl Freter. Lastly, a heartfelt thank-you to all of the laboratory personnel who were so graciously helpful in preparing and obtaining the blood smears and bone marrow aspirates for the past four decades. Without them, this book would never have been possible.

CONTENTS

A 74-year-old male with no significant medical history is referred by his primary care physician for further evaluation of generalized lymphadenopathy. Patient reports no preceding weight loss, night sweats, or fever. On physical examination, lymphadenopathy and splenomegaly are found, with the spleen edge palpable 7 cm below the left costal margin. Laboratory workup reveals a total leukocyte count of 36,500/μL, with the majority of cells of the type shown below, hemoglobin 14.5 g/dL and a platelet count of 342,000/μL.

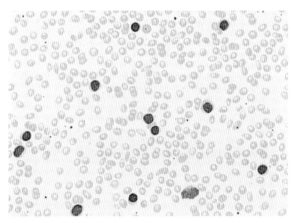
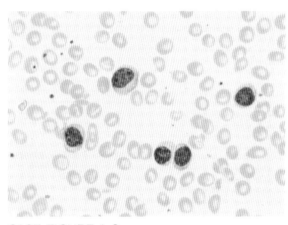

CASE FIGURE 1-1   CASE FIGURE 1-2

QUESTION 1

✯ What is the most likely diagnosis based on clinical presentation and peripheral blood smear findings?

A. Mantle cell lymphoma (MCL)

B. Follicular lymphoma (FL)

C. Acute myeloid leukemia (AML)

D. Small lymphocytic lymphoma (SLL)

E. Chronic lymphocytic leukemia (CLL)

Answer: E. The blood smear shows a major population of small lymphocytes with condensed chromatin and a "smudge cell." The patient's presentation with generalized asymptomatic lymphadenopathy and splenomegaly and increased small mature lymphocytes as depicted in the blood smear is most consistent with the diagnosis of CLL, which is the most common type of leukemia in the Western world. Statistically, CLL would be the most likely diagnosis. SLL is considered a nodal counterpart of CLL and is diagnosed when lymphadenopathy is present and the peripheral blood monoclonal B lymphocyte count is less than 5,000/μL. CLL requires the presence of at least 5,000 monoclonal B lymphocytes per μL. Cases not meeting diagnostic criteria for SLL with less than 5,000 monoclonal B lymphocytes per μL in peripheral blood, with otherwise typical flow cytometry features of CLL, are denoted as clonal B-cell lymphocytosis (*Blood*. 2008;111(12):5446).

QUESTION 2

✵ What is the typical flow cytometric pattern seen in cases of CLL?

A. CD5–, CD10+, CD19–, CD20+, CD23+

B. CD5+, CD19+, CD20+, CD23–

C. CD5+, CD19+, CD20+, CD23+

D. CD5–, CD19+, CD20+, CD23+

E. CD5–, CD19+, CD20+, CD23–

Answer: C. CLL is characterized by expression of CD5, CD19, CD20 (dim), and CD23. Positivity for CD23 differentiates it from MCL, which is typically negative for CD23, and positivity for CD5 differentiates it from other B-cell non-Hodgkin lymphomas (*Blood*. 2008;111(12):5446).

QUESTION 3

✵ What is the most common cytogenetic abnormality detected in CLL?

A. 17p deletion

B. 11q deletion

C. Trisomy 12

D. 13q deletion

E. 6q

Answer: D. Chromosomal abnormalities are detected in 82% of CLL cases. Deletion 13q is seen in 45% to 55% of cases, deletion 11q in 18% to 20%, trisomy 12 in 15% to 16%, deletion 6q in 7%, and deletion 17p in 7% to 10% of de novo CLL cases (*N Engl J Med*. 2000;343(26):1910, *Blood*. 1997;89(7):2516). In addition, SF3B1 and other novel cancer genes have been reported in CLL. SF3B1 has been noted primarily with deletion 11q cases and is associated with a poor prognosis (*N Engl J Med*. 2011;365:2497–2506).

QUESTION 4

✵ Patient was found to have deletion 13q, and after a 23-month observation period the patient presented for follow-up with increased lymphadenopathy. Patient also reported a 1-month history of night sweats in addition to a 20-pound weight loss. What would be the most appropriate therapeutic regimen?

A. Cyclophosphamide, doxorubicin, vincristine, prednisone, rituximab (CHOP-R)

B. Cyclophosphamide, vincristine, prednisone, rituximab (CVP-R)

C. Cyclophosphamide (C)

D. Fludarabine, cyclophosphamide, rituximab (FCR)

E. Chlorambucil

Answer: D. Fludarabine-based regimens (FC, FR, FCR) are considered standard of care for first-line treatment of de novo CLL. Bendamustine–rituximab (BR) would also be an appropriate regimen.

QUESTION 5

Patient received 4 cycles of FCR with significant decrease in the size of lymph nodes, normalization of lymphocyte count, and disappearance of B symptoms. Five months after completion of therapy, patient presented to the emergency department complaining of subacute change in his mental status. Complete blood count revealed normal peripheral blood counts. After a negative computed tomography (CT) scan of the head, cerebrospinal fluid (CSF) analysis was performed with increased levels of protein, normal glucose levels, and increased lymphocyte counts. Microscopic examination of CSF is shown below.

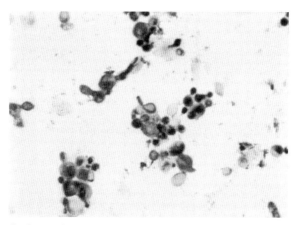

CASE FIGURE 1-3

✶ What is the most likely diagnosis based on the clinical presentation and CSF examination?

A. Meningeal leukemia

B. Hyperleukocytosis

C. Cryptococcal meningitis

D. Cerebrovascular accident

E. Streptococcal meningitis

Answer: C. Cryptococcal organisms are noted in the CSF as translucent "soap bubbles" among an inflammatory infiltrate, and stain positive with India ink. Antigen testing for *Cryptococcus* was also positive. Fludarabine-induced lymphopenia increases the risk of opportunistic infections, and prophylactic anti-infective agents should be considered during, and for several months after, completion of fludarabine-based therapy (*Am J Hematol.* 1995;49(2):135).

QUESTION 6

Patient was appropriately treated for cryptococcal meningitis with resolution of neurological symptoms. However, 18 months after completion of initial therapy, patient presented with recurrence of night sweats and 15-pound weight loss. Laboratory evaluation revealed a lymphocyte count of 112,000/μL. Peripheral blood smear is shown below.

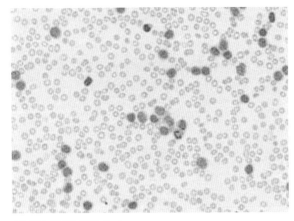

CASE FIGURE 1-4

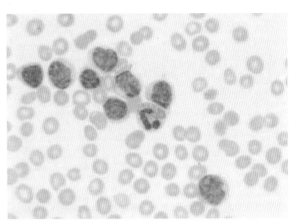

CASE FIGURE 1-5

✮ What is the most likely explanation for his clinical presentation?

A. Transformation to acute lymphoblastic leukemia

B. Prolymphocytic transformation

C. Richter syndrome

D. Disseminated cryptococcal infection

E. Fludarabine-induced myelodysplastic syndrome

Answer: B. Peripheral slide reveals a combination of the typical small lymphocytes characteristic of CLL, in addition to larger lymphocytes, with a prominent single nucleolus, less condensed chromatin, and more abundant cytoplasm. Clinical presentation is most consistent with prolymphocytic transformation, which develops in 10% of CLL cases and usually represents a terminal event secondary to resistance to usual chemotherapeutic agents. Richter transformation occurs in less than 10% of cases and refers to progression to an aggressive form of NHL (*Cancer.* 1981;48(11):2447, *Br J Haematol.* 1986;64(1):77).

QUESTION 7

✮ What would be an appropriate therapeutic regimen at this time given the new clinical development?

A. Single-agent rituximab

B. Chlorambucil

C. Allogeneic hematopoietic stem cell transplantation (HSCT)

D. Alemtuzumab

E. Retreatment with FCR

Answer: D. Alemtuzumab has modest activity in cases of prolymphocytic transformation. Retreatment with FCR can be considered if no other options are available. Allogeneic HSCT is unlikely to be an option, given patient's advanced age (*Leuk Lymphoma*. 2002;43(5):1007).

CASE 2

A 21-year-old African American male is referred by his primary care physician for further evaluation of anemia. Patient denies history of melena or hematochezia. There is no prior history of episodic bone pain or family history of blood disorders. Physical examination reveals a young male with no hepatosplenomegaly. Laboratory workup reveals a total leukocyte count of 6,500/μL, hemoglobin 7.2 g/dL, mean corpuscular volume (MCV) 67 fL, red blood cell count of 2.2 million/μL, and platelet count of 280,000/μL. Peripheral blood smear is shown below.

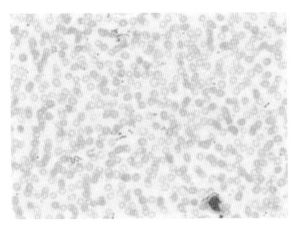

CASE FIGURE 2-1

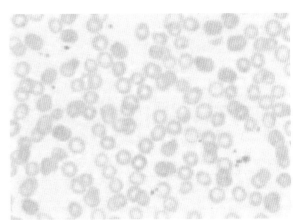

CASE FIGURE 2-2

QUESTION 1

✭ What is the most likely diagnosis?

A. Beta thalassemia major
B. Alpha thalassemia trait
C. Iron-deficiency anemia
D. Beta sickle cell thalassemia
E. Beta thalassemia intermedia

Answer: C. The blood smear shows microcytic hypochromic red cells without basophilic stippling. Iron-deficiency anemia is characterized by microcytic hypochromic red blood cells. Microcytosis would be expected in beta thalassemia intermedia or major as well as in alpha thalassemia trait.

However, a decreased red blood cell count is more consistent with iron deficiency, as thalassemic disorders typically present with microcytic polycythemia, and basophilic stippling may be seen in the red cells. In addition to iron deficiency and thalassemic disorders including hemoglobin C, D, and E diseases, differential diagnosis of microcytic anemia includes anemia of chronic disease, congenital sideroblastic anemia, lead poisoning, aluminum toxicity associated with dialysis, copper deficiency, zinc excess, and hereditary pyropoikilocytosis. Iron deficiency is always a manifestation of an underlying pathologic process, and evaluation should always proceed to uncover the underlying disease entity.

QUESTION 2

On further questioning, the patient reported several month history of hemoptysis; however, he denied hematuria, epistaxis, or a sore throat. Chest x-ray revealed bilateral interstitial and hilar infiltrates (shown below). Urine analysis showed microscopic hematuria. Lung biopsy was obtained with evidence of hemosiderin-laden macrophages.

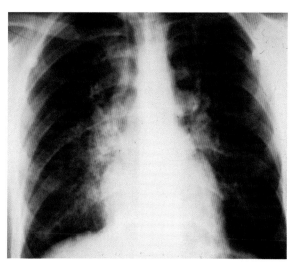

CASE FIGURE 2-3

☆ What is the most likely underlying diagnosis?

A. Streptococcal pneumonia

B. Mitral valve prolapse

C. Pulmonary embolism

D. Goodpasture syndrome

E. Wegener granulomatosis

Answer: D. Goodpasture syndrome is associated with pulmonary vasculitis and nephritic syndrome. It is caused by pathologic autoantibodies directed against collagen type IV in the glomerular basement membrane as well as pulmonary vasculature. Wegener granulomatosis is associated with involvement of the upper respiratory tracts in addition to pulmonary and renal vasculature. Antineutrophil cytoplasmic antibodies directed against proteinase 3 are typically detected in Wegener granulomatosis (*Ann Intern Med.* 1996;124(7):651).

CASE 3

A 48-year-old male presents to the emergency room for further evaluation of a 3-week history of progressively worsening fatigue. Physical examination reveals pallor and diffuse petechiae over lower extremities. Laboratory evaluation shows a total leukocyte count of 23,400/μL, hemoglobin 9.8 g/dL, and platelet count of 13,000/μL. Peripheral blood smear and bone marrow aspirate are shown.

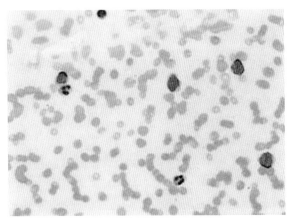

CASE FIGURE 3-1

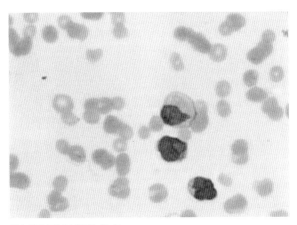

CASE FIGURE 3-2

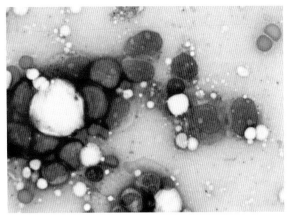

CASE FIGURE 3-3

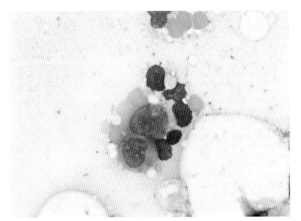

CASE FIGURE 3-4

QUESTION 1

✯ What is the most likely diagnosis?

A. Acute lymphoblastic leukemia (ALL)

B. Acute myeloid leukemia (AML)

C. Prolymphocytic leukemia (PLL)

D. Chronic myeloid leukemia (CML)

E. Chronic lymphocytic leukemia (CLL)

Answer: B. Peripheral slide demonstrates large leukocytes with fine, uncondensed chromatin structure with high nuclear to cytoplasmic ratio characteristic of blasts. The presence of Auer rods is pathognomonic of acute myeloid leukemia. A bone marrow aspirate disclosed 36% blasts with salmon granules and a perinuclear hof. Fluorescence in situ hybridization (FISH) revealed t(8;21). AML with t(8;21) results in the fusion of RUNX1 and RUNX1T1, which disrupts function of the core binding factor. AML t(8;21) accounts for about 8% of AML and is associated with a favorable prognosis.

QUESTION 2

✯ What is the typical flow cytometry pattern of an AML?

A. CD13+, CD33−, CD34−, HLD-DR+

B. CD13+, CD33+, CD34+, HLD-DR+

C. CD13−, CD33+, CD34−, HLD-DR−

D. CD13−, CD33−, CD34−, HLD-DR+

E. CD13+, CD33+, CD34−, HLD-DR+

Answer: B. The typical flow cytometry pattern of AML includes positivity for CD13, CD33, CD34, and HLA-DR. APL is typically negative for CD34 and HLD-DR, which can serve as a quick and simple diagnostic tool (*Arch Pathol Lab Med.* 2003;127(1):42, *Blood.* 2008;111(8):3941).

QUESTION 3

✯ Which of the following scenarios meets the current WHO criteria for the diagnosis of AML?

A. Bone marrow blast count of 8% with deletion 5q

B. Bone marrow blast count of 16% with monosomy 7

C. Bone marrow blast count of 6% with translocation t(8;21)

D. Bone marrow blast count of 12% with translocation t(9;22)

E. Bone marrow blast count of 18% with translocation t(8;14)

Answer: C. The current WHO criteria defines AML as the presence of 20% or more blasts in the bone marrow or peripheral blood or the presence of any of the following chromosomal abnormalities regardless of the blast count, t(8;21), t(16;16), inv(16), t(15;17) (*Blood.* 2009;114(5):937).

QUESTION 4

☆ Which of the following defines a poor prognostic criterion as defined by cytogenetic abnormalities?

A. t(8;21)

B. t(16;16)

C. t(9;11)

D. t(15;17)

E. t(14;18)

Answer: C. t(8;21), t(16;16), inv(16), and t(15;17) define a favorable risk group of AML. Translocation t(9;11) usually involves the MLL gene located at 11q23 and is associated with a poor prognosis. Translocation t(14;18) is seen in the majority of follicular lymphoma (FL) cases; however, it is not diagnostic of FL as it can be found in multiple other lymphoma subtypes (*Blood.* 2010;116(3):354).

QUESTION 5

☆ Which of the following genetic abnormalities defines a favorable prognosis group?

A. FLT3-ITD+, NPM1+

B. Monoallelic CEBPA+, FLT3-ITD−

C. NPM1+, FLT3-ITD−

D. Biallelic CEBPA+, FLT3-ITD+

E. NPM1−, FLT3-ITD−

Answer: C. Presence of NPM1 mutation confers favorable prognosis in AML patients with normal cytogenetics, while FLT3-ITD is associated with poor outcomes. The presence of biallelic mutations in CEBPA is associated with a favorable mutation. Monoallelic CEBPA mutations do not appear to predict the same favorable outcome (*Blood.* 2011;118(4):1069, *Blood.* 2011;118(20):5593, *Blood.* 2010;115(3):453).

QUESTION 6

☆ Presence of which of the following is associated with worse outcomes in patients with AML bearing t(8;21)?

A. t(8;14)

B. KIT D816V mutation

C. JAK2 V617F mutation

D. t(11;14)

E. Hyperdiploidy

Answer: B. Presence of KIT D816V mutation is associated with a negative outlook in patients with core-binding factor AML harboring t(8;21), t(16;16), or inv(16), otherwise classified in the favorable prognosis group. This mutation has been reported in 30% to 40% of adults and increases the relapse rate from 30% to 70% (*J Clin Oncol.* 2006;34(24):3904, *Br J Haematol.* 2010;148(6):925).

QUESTION 7

☆ Patient achieved a complete remission following induction chemotherapy. What is the most appropriate management following achievement of complete remission?

A. Observation

B. Refer for autologous HSCT

C. Refer for allogeneic HSCT

D. Consolidation with high-dose cytarabine

E. Consolidation with 5 days of cytarabine with 2 days of daunorubicin

Answer: D. Patients younger than 60 years of age with favorable cytogenetic profile appear to derive survival benefit from repeated cycles of high-dose cytarabine consolidation. There does not appear to be benefit for allogeneic HSCT in first remission in such patient population. Contrastingly, high-risk patients should be referred for allogeneic HSCT after achieving first remission. There is no role for autologous HSCT in the management of AML (*N Engl J Med.* 1994;331(14):896, *JAMA.* 2009;301(22):2349, *Cancer.* 2005;103(8):1652).

CASE 4

A 74-year-old female presents for evaluation of chronic and progressive fatigue and weakness. She lives with two cats and a German Shepherd dog. Patient has a history of hypertension and hyperlipidemia with occasional gastroesophageal reflux symptoms. Patient reports no prior surgical procedures. Urine analysis reveals no evidence of hematuria or hemoglobinuria. Stool is negative for occult blood. Laboratory evaluation reveals hemoglobin of 4.2 g/dL, mean corpuscular volume (MCV) of 120 fL, leukocyte count of 2,100/μL, platelet count of 45,000/μL, and an LDH level of 4,700 U/L. Peripheral blood smear is shown.

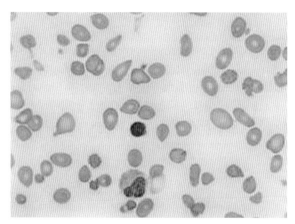

CASE FIGURE 4-1

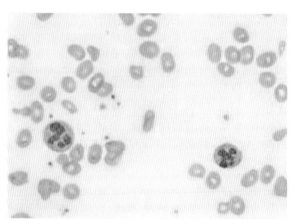

CASE FIGURE 4-2

QUESTION 1

✹ Which of the following is not among the possible explanations of the patient's presentation?

A. Folic acid deficiency

B. Hereditary elliptocytosis

C. Hemolytic anemia

D. Liver disease

E. Medication use

Answer: B. Hereditary elliptocytosis would not explain patient's pancytopenia, macrocytosis, and hypersegmented neutrophils, as noted in the above images of the peripheral blood. Differential diagnosis of macrocytosis includes vitamin B12 and folate deficiency; liver disease; hypothyroidism; medication use such as trimethoprim-sulfamethoxazole, methotrexate, and cytotoxic chemotherapy; reticulocytosis; myelodysplastic syndromes; excessive alcohol use; and aplastic anemia.

QUESTION 2

✭ Further evaluation revealed vitamin B12 level 292 pg/mL, serum folate 0.9 ng/mL, and RBC folate 24 ng/mL. Methylmalonic acid level was normal, while homocysteine was found to be elevated. What is the most likely diagnosis?

A. Folic acid deficiency

B. Vitamin B12 deficiency

C. Combined folic acid and vitamin B12 deficiency

Answer: A. Decreased levels of serum and RBC folate in conjunction with normal levels of methylmalonic acid are consistent with the diagnosis of folic acid deficiency. Elevation of both methylmalonic acid and homocysteine can be used to detect cases of early vitamin B12 deficiency, as methylmalonic acid levels are normal in folic acid deficiency, while homocysteine is usually elevated. RBC folate levels are considered to be a better reflection of tissue folate stores compared with serum folate, which can fluctuate widely following meals. However, studies have shown that the information provided by both tests is comparable, and thus the more expensive RBC folate test is reserved for cases of high suspicion for folate deficiency despite normal serum folate levels. The methylfolate trap hypothesis predicts higher serum folate levels in conjunction with lower RBC folate levels associated with vitamin B12 deficiency, as reduced methionine synthase activity causes reduced intracellular methylfolate metabolism and slow cellular loss by diffusion into the circulation. However, this hypothesis has never been definitely demonstrated in humans (*J Clin Pathol.* 2003;56(12):924, *Br J Haematol.* 2006;132(5):623).

CASE 5

A 66-year-old female previously healthy presents for further evaluation of diffuse bone pain, left-sided abdominal discomfort, and progressive fatigue for the last several months. Examination is significant for splenomegaly, easily palpable below the left costal margin extending to the midline. Laboratory evaluation reveals leukocyte count of 167,000/μL, hemoglobin 9.2 g/dL, and platelet count of 730,000/μL. Peripheral blood smear is shown.

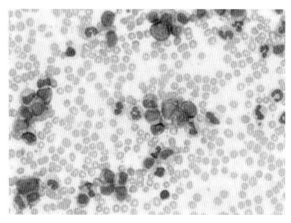

CASE FIGURE 5-1

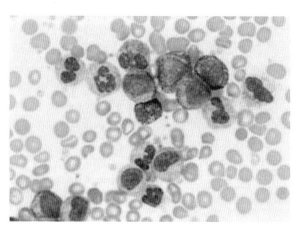

CASE FIGURE 5-2

QUESTION 1

✩ What is the most likely diagnosis based on this clinical presentation?

A. Chronic lymphocytic leukemia (CLL)
B. Acute myeloid leukemia (AML)
C. Chronic myeloid leukemia (CML)
D. Acute lymphocytic leukemia (ALL)
E. Hairy cell leukemia (HCL)

Answer: C. The typical peripheral blood picture of chronic phase CML reveals evidence of left-shifted myeloid leukocytes with increased numbers of mature neutrophils, bands, myelocytes, and promyelocytes with little or no peripheral blasts. In addition, absolute basophilia is always present, usually with eosinophilia, as noted in the images. AML and ALL would be expected to exhibit increased number of myeloid or lymphoid blasts, respectively, in peripheral blood. CLL is characterized by increased numbers of mature lymphocytes in peripheral blood. HCL typically presents with pancytopenia, and monocytopenia is very commonly seen and is a useful clue to the diagnosis.

QUESTION 2

Bone marrow biopsy is obtained with evidence of increased marrow cellularity and expanded myeloid lineages as shown below.

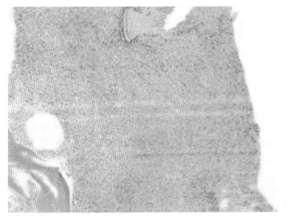

CASE FIGURE 5-3   CASE FIGURE 5-4

✫ What is the expected chromosomal abnormality?

A. t(9;21)

B. t(14;18)

C. t(8;14)

D. t(9;22)

E. t(9;11)

Answer: D. Philadelphia chromosome (Ph chromosome) resulting from t(9;22) creates a chimeric fusion gene *BCR-ABL*. The presence and expression of *BCR-ABL* is the defining feature of CML, as well as the underlying pathophysiologic abnormality of CML. Ph chromosome resulting from t(9;22) is detected in 90% to 95% of cases, and the remaining 5% to 10% are referred to as Ph-negative CML. These cases of Ph-negative CML have cryptic translocations that cannot be detected by cytogenetics and require FISH or PCR for identification (*Cancer Genet Cytogenet.* 2007;173(2):97, *Br J Haematol.* 2004;125(2):187).

QUESTION 3

Patient is started on imatinib 400 mg daily and is seen for follow-up 1 month later. Evaluation reveals near-complete normalization of peripheral blood counts. However, patient reports progressively worsening dyspnea on exertion, in addition to periorbital and distal lower extremity swelling. Chest x-ray is shown below.

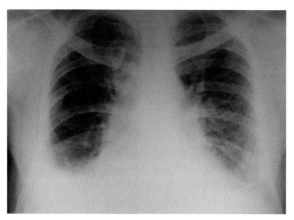

CASE FIGURE 5-5

☆ What is the most likely etiology of patient's most recent presentation?

A. Leukostasis
B. Interstitial lung disease
C. Leukemic infiltration
D. Fluid overload
E. Heart failure

Answer: D. Fluid overload manifesting as pulmonary edema, peripheral edema, and periorbital edema is a relatively common side effect of BCR-ABL inhibitors and is thought to be related to inhibition of platelet-derived growth factor receptor, resulting in increased capillary-to-interstitium transport. Leukostasis or leukemic infiltration would be less likely, given the near normalization of peripheral blood counts. Heart failure and interstitial lung disease have been rarely reported with imatinib; however, the acute presentation is more consistent with imatinib-induced fluid overload (*Cancer Res.* 2001;61(7):2929).

QUESTION 4

Imatinib is temporarily discontinued, and the patient is treated with diuretics. Imatinib is reintroduced with no further recurrence of periorbital edema. Patient continues on imatinib for the next 3 years and achieves complete molecular response by 18 months. However, 46 months after initiation of therapy, she presents complaining of several months of worsening fatigue, left-sided abdominal pain, and night sweats. Patient reports adherence to imatinib regimen. Evaluation reveals leukocyte count of 125,000/μL, hemoglobin 8.2 g/dL, and platelet count of 80,000/μL. Peripheral blood smear is shown below.

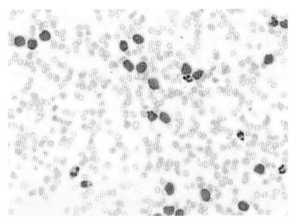

CASE FIGURE 5-6

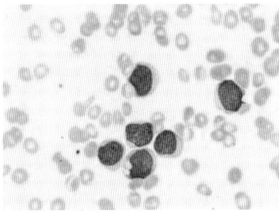

CASE FIGURE 5-7

★ What is the most likely explanation of her presentation?

A. Imatinib toxicity
B. Transformation to chronic lymphocytic leukemia
C. Progression to acute myeloid leukemia
D. Development of myelofibrosis
E. Noncompliance with imatinib

Answer: C. Medication noncompliance should always be considered in the differential diagnosis of a CML patient with suboptimal response or loss of response to therapy. However, in this case patient reports adherence to her regimen, which makes this a less likely etiology. Peripheral smear reveals predominance of a uniform cell population with increased nuclear-to-cytoplasmic ratio with fine chromatin consistent with myeloblasts. Bone marrow aspirate showed 64% myeloblasts. This picture is diagnostic of progression to AML.

CASE 6

A 32-year-old female is found on routine physical examination to have splenomegaly. She reports no acute change in her energy levels. However, she does note being more easily fatigued during heavy physical activity as long as she can remember. Patient reports a history of cholelithiasis diagnosed 10 years previously; however, she elected not to undergo cholecystectomy. Mild splenomegaly is noted on physical examination. Laboratory workup reveals hemoglobin 11.2 g/dL, mean corpuscular volume (MCV) 85 fL, leukocyte count 6,500/μL, and platelet count of 361,000/μL. Indirect bilirubin level is minimally elevated, and the direct antiglobin test is negative. Peripheral blood smear is shown below.

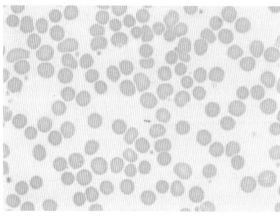

CASE FIGURE 6-1

QUESTION 1

☆ What is the most likely diagnosis?

A. Iron-deficiency anemia
B. Beta thalassemia intermedia
C. Hereditary spherocytosis (HS)
D. Autoimmune hemolytic anemia (AIHA)
E. Anemia of chronic disease

Answer: C. Peripheral blood smear reveals a single population of red blood cells (RBC) with no central pallor zone consistent with spherocytes. Patient's prior history of cholelithiasis at a young age and normal mean corpuscular volume (MCV) and normal other blood lineages, in addition to spleno-megaly, is consistent with a diagnosis of hereditary spherocytosis with chronic mild hemolytic anemia. Negative direct antiglobin test makes the diagnosis of AIHA unlikely. Normal MCV argues strongly against beta thalassemia intermedia.

QUESTION 2

✮ What is the underlying molecular defect in hereditary spherocytosis?

A. Defects in the vertical interactions between membrane skeleton and the lipid bilayer

B. Defects in the horizontal interactions between membrane skeleton and the lipid bilayer

C. Defective ion transport across red blood cell membrane

D. Defective ability to neutralize oxidative stress

E. Abnormal hemoglobin polymers causing red blood cell membrane damage

Answer: A. Hereditary spherocytosis is caused by defects in the vertical interactions between membrane skeleton and the lipid bilayer secondary to functional deficiency or absence of spectrin, ankyrin, protein 4.2, and band 3. Hereditary elliptocytosis is caused by defects in the horizontal interactions. Hereditary spherocytosis classically presents as a mild to moderate hemolytic anemia with variable degrees of splenomegaly (*Br J Haematol*. 1999;104(1):2).

QUESTION 3

✮ What would be the most sensitive and specific test to confirm the diagnosis?

A. Osmotic fragility test

B. Cryohemolysis test

C. Eosin-5-maleimide binding test (EMA)

D. Incubation of red blood cells with diepoxybutane (DEB)

E. Spleen biopsy

Answer: C. EMA testing is a flow cytometry-based test which provides a rapid diagnosis of HS with minimal volume of required red blood cells. Sensitivity and specificity are much higher compared with other available tests and are reported to be 92.7% and 99.1%, respectively. The sensitivity and specific-ity of osmotic fragility testing is considerably lower at 68% to 81% (*Haematologica*. 2012;97(4):516, *Br J Haematol*. 2000;111(3):924).

QUESTION 4

Patient underwent splenectomy with normalization in her hemoglobin level. Two years after the procedure, she presents to the emergency department with acute onset of fever, confusion, and hypotension refractory to aggressive intravenous fluid adminis-tration. Laboratory evaluation reveals pancytopenia with acute renal failure. Blood cul-tures returns positive for Gram-negative bacteria as shown below. Peripheral blood smear and bone marrow aspirate are reviewed and are shown below.

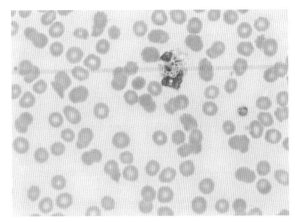

CASE FIGURE 6-2

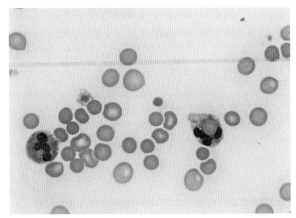

CASE FIGURE 6-3

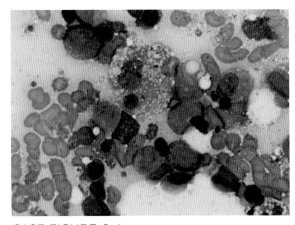

CASE FIGURE 6-4

☆ What is the most likely explanation for her clinical presentation?

A. Autoimmune hemolytic anemia with immune thrombocytopenia

B. Gram-negative sepsis with multiorgan failure

C. Hemophagocytic syndrome

D. Acute myeloid leukemia

E. Thrombotic thrombocytopenic purpura

Answer: C. Peripheral blood smear reveals erythrophagocytosis, and bone marrow aspirate shows hemophagocytosis. This blood smear picture, in addition to her presentation with pancytopenia and Gram-negative sepsis in a postsplenectomy setting, is most consistent with secondary hemophagocytic syndrome associated with bacterial infection. Answer B is partially correct, however, as it does not explain the peripheral blood picture and bone marrow images (*Cancer.* 1984;54(12):2968).

A 67-year-old male presents for further evaluation secondary to persistent bleeding from a hyperpigmented lesion on the hard palate that had been biopsied 5 days previously (shown below).

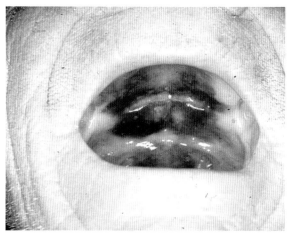

CASE FIGURE 7-1

Patient reports having good health with no significant prior medical history. Evaluation reveals leukocyte count of 2,100/μL, ANC 800/μL, hemoglobin of 8.2/dL, and platelet count of 82,000/μL. PT and PTT are prolonged. Images of the peripheral blood smear and bone marrow aspirate are shown below.

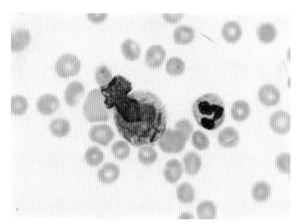

CASE FIGURE 7-2

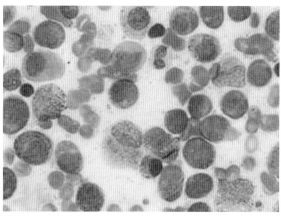

CASE FIGURE 7-3

QUESTION 1

✫ What is the most likely diagnosis?

A. Acute lymphocytic leukemia (ALL)

B. Acute myeloid leukemia (AML)

C. Acute promyelocytic leukemia (APL)

D. Thrombotic thrombocytopenic purpura (TTP)

E. Sepsis

Answer: C. The peripheral blood smear shows a hypergranular leukocyte with multiple Auer rods ("faggot cell"), while the bone marrow reveals increased promyelocytes with numerous cytoplasmic granules, and a few cells exhibit multiple Auer rods. This presentation with bleeding, pancytopenia, coagulation abnormalities, and the presence of multiple Auer rods is highly suspicious for hypergranular acute promyelocytic leukemia (APL). FISH for t(15;17) was positive and hence confirmed a diagnosis of hypergranular APL. APL constitutes 5% to 8% of AML, and the hypergranular variant accounts for 60% to 70% of cases and usually presents with leukopenia. The t(15;17) results in the fusion of the PML gene with the retinoic acid receptor (RARA) gene. APL is a specific subclass of AML classified as AML with t(15;17) by the WHO classification and as AML-M3 under the old FAB classification (*Br J Haematol.* 2012;156(1):24).

QUESTION 2

✫ What are the characteristic flow cytometric findings in APL?

A. CD13+, CD33+, CD34+, HLA-DR–

B. CD13+, CD33–, CD34+, HLA-DR–

C. CD13+, CD33+, CD34–, HLA-DR–

D. CD13–, CD33–, CD34–, HLA-DR+

E. CD13+, CD33+, CD34+, HLA-DR+

Answer: C. Contrasting with other subtypes of AML, APL is characteristically negative for CD34 and HLA-DR. This can provide a quick and early clue to the underlying diagnosis (*Blood.* 2009;113(9):1875).

QUESTION 3

Treatment is initiated with all-trans-retinoic acid (ATRA) and daunorubicin. Ten days later, the patient reports worsening dyspnea, cough, fever, and lower extremity swelling. Laboratory evaluation reveals leukocyte count of 17,800/µL. Chest x-ray is obtained and is shown below.

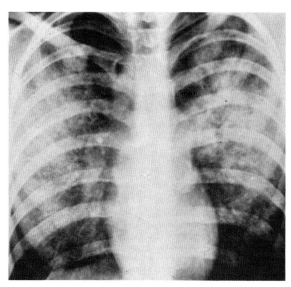

CASE FIGURE 7-4

✯ What would be the next most appropriate step in the management of this patient?

A. Diuresis

B. Echocardiogram

C. Infectious workup and initiation of broad-spectrum antibiotics

D. Infectious workup and initiation of dexamethasone

E. Reinduction with daunorubicin, cytarabine, and arsenic trioxide (ATO)

Answer: D. Presentation is most consistent with APL differentiation syndrome that can be associated with the use of ATRA or ATO. Prompt initiation of dexamethasone is considered the treatment of choice, and temporary discontinuation of ATRA or ATO can be considered in the most severe cases pending improvement. APL differentiation syndrome presents with fever, hypoxemia, pulmonary infiltrates, hypotension, renal dysfunction, edema, and weight gain, which can mimic sepsis. Infectious workup is indicated to rule out an underlying infection (*Blood.* 2009;113(4):775, *Blood.* 2000;95(1):90).

A 60-year-old female with a history of hypertension and hyperlipidemia presents in December for further evaluation of several months history of generalized fatigue. Patient denies bleeding, weight loss, or changes in appetite. Physical examination reveals no jaundice, lymphadenopathy, or organomegaly. Laboratory evaluation shows hemoglobin of 8.7 g/dL, mean corpuscular volume (MCV) of 110 fL, leukocyte count of 5,600/μL, and platelet count of 174,000/μL. Peripheral blood smear is shown below.

CASE FIGURE 8-1

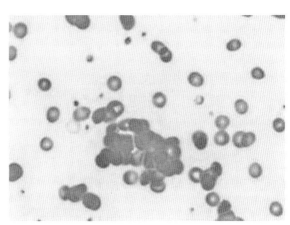

CASE FIGURE 8-2

QUESTION 1

☆ What is the most likely diagnosis based on the clinical presentation and peripheral blood smear?

A. Autoimmune hemolytic anemia

B. Reticulocytosis

C. Liver disease

D. Multiple myeloma

E. Cold agglutinin disease

Answer: E. Peripheral slide reveals areas of red blood cells (RBC) clumping, which result in a spurious elevation of MCV. Patient's presentation is consistent with cold agglutinin disease, which is characterized by the presence of IgM antibodies directed against I antigen on the surface of RBCs. Abnormal antibodies react with RBC at less than physiologic body temperatures and result in hemolytic anemia. High titer of cold agglutinins is used to confirm the diagnosis. Warming of the blood, as depicted below, results in disappearance of RBC agglutination. Cold agglutinin disease can be related to underlying infections, such as mycoplasma, EBV, CMV or hepatitis virus, lymphoproliferative disorders, connective tissue disease, or other autoimmune disorders or may be idiopathic.

CASE FIGURE 8-3

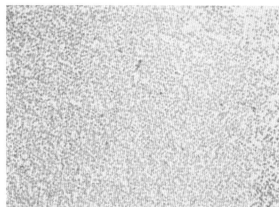

CASE FIGURE 8-4

QUESTION 2

✲ What are the most likely findings on direct antiglobin test?

A. Negative for IgG and complement

B. Positive for complement only

C. Positive for IgG and complement

D. Positive for IgG only

Answer: B. Washing of the RBCs during direct antiglobin test results in dissociation of abnormal antibodies from the surface of RBCs. This leaves only complement attached to the RBC surface. Since the majority of cold agglutinin disease cases are caused by a pathologic IgM, testing for IgG will produce negative results. In the rare case of IgG cold agglutinin disease, poor fixation of abnormal antibody to the surface of the RBC might result in its dissociation and removal during RBC washing, leaving only complement.

QUESTION 3

Patient is counseled to avoid cold exposure, and on a follow-up visit 2 months later, her hemoglobin is 10.8 g/dL. In August, patient presents to the emergency department with recurrent fatigue and is found to have a hemoglobin of 7.2 g/dL. Patient denies recent infections. On examination, no lymphadenopathy or organomegaly are detected. CT scan is performed with no evidence of underlying malignancy.

✭ What is the most appropriate management to control her disease at this time?

A. Corticosteroids

B. Intravenous immunoglobulins (IVIG)

C. Rituximab

D. Cyclophosphamide, vincristine, prednisone, rituximab (CVP-R)

E. Splenectomy

Answer: C. Rituximab should be considered the treatment of choice. Although corticosteroids are effective in the management of warm autoimmune hemolytic anemia, they do not have a role in the management of cold agglutinin disease. IVIG infusions are also without significant benefits. Splenectomy is unlikely to provide clinical benefit as the spleen is not the site of hemolysis. Rituximab has been shown to induce remissions either alone or when used in combination with other agents; however, the additional toxicity provided by a combination cytotoxic regimen is not justified at this time. Plasma exchange has been used as a means to rapidly remove the abnormal antibody from the circulation; however, the benefits of this procedure are short lived (*Br J Haematol.* 2007;138(4):422, *Blood.* 2010;116(17):3180, *Br J Haematol.* 2011;153(3):309, *Blood.* 2012;119(16):3691).

A 70-year-old male with prior medical history of diabetes and hypertension is referred by his primary care physician for further evaluation of elevated leukocyte count, anemia, and thrombocytopenia. The patient initially presented to his primary care physician secondary to a 3-week history of progressive rash on his face, as shown below.

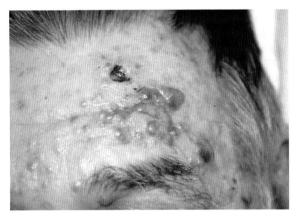

CASE FIGURE 9-1

Laboratory values reveals a leukocyte count of 57,000/μL, hemoglobin of 8.2 g/dL, and platelets of 43,000/μL. Peripheral blood smear and skin lesion biopsy are shown below.

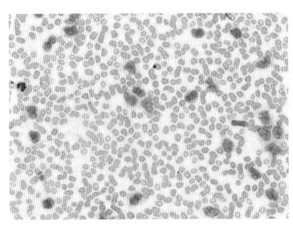

CASE FIGURE 9-2

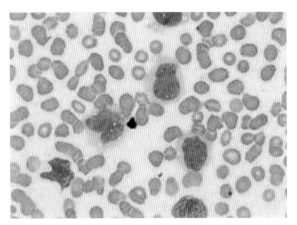

CASE FIGURE 9-3

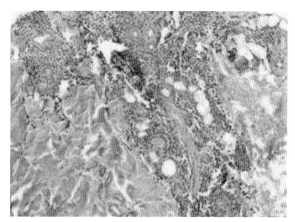

CASE FIGURE 9-4

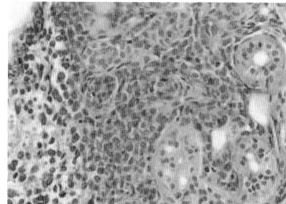

CASE FIGURE 9-5

QUESTION 1

✲ What is the most likely diagnosis?

A. Acute lymphocytic leukemia

B. Acute monoblastic leukemia

C. Chronic myeloid leukemia

D. Chronic lymphocytic leukemia

E. Peripheral T-cell lymphoma

Answer: B. Peripheral blood smear reveals increased number of myeloid blasts exhibiting mono-cytic features. Skin biopsy demonstrates infiltration by a monotonous cell population. The clinical presentation is most consistent with acute monoblastic leukemia (AML-M5 by FAB classification) and was confirmed by flow cytometry (CD13, CD33, CD14, CD68 positive). Leukemia cutis presents in approximately 3% of cases of AML (*Ann Hematol.* 2002;81(2):90); however, it is seen in up to 50% of cases of myelomonocytic and monocytic differentiation (*Blood.* 1980;55(1):71, *Blood.* 2011; 118(14):3785).

QUESTION 2

✲ What is the most commonly associated cytogenetic abnormality?

A. t(8;21)

B. t(9;11)

C. inv(16)

D. t(6;9)

E. inv(3)

Answer: B. t(9;11) involving rearrangement of 11q23 have been associated with acute monoblastic leukemia (*Leuk Res.* 1982;6(1):17, *Blood.* 1986;67(2):484).

CASE 10

A 36-year-old African American male presents for further evaluation of mild anemia. Patient reports feeling well and is active in several types of sports with no limitation. There is no history of bleeding or episodic bone pain. Physical examination reveals no hepatosplenomegaly or lymphadenopathy. Laboratory evaluation reveals hemoglobin level of 12.1 g/dL, mean corpuscular volume (MCV) of 62 fL, red blood cell count of 6,100,000/μL, and platelet count of 254,000/μL. Hemoglobin electrophoresis was performed and revealed a normal pattern. Peripheral smear is shown below.

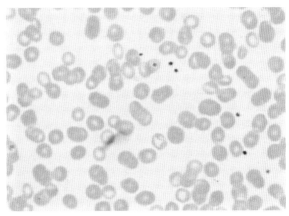

CASE FIGURE 10-1

QUESTION 1

★ What is the most likely diagnosis?

A. Alpha thalassemia silent carrier

B. Beta thalassemia trait

C. Alpha thalassemia trait

D. Beta thalassemia intermedia

E. Iron-deficiency anemia

Answer: C. Alpha thalassemia trait results from a deletion of 2 alpha globin genes. The clinical phenotype is that of mild hypochromic microcytic anemia in an asymptomatic or minimally symptomatic individual. Hemoglobin electrophoresis is typically normal in contrast to increased HbA2 fraction seen in cases of beta thalassemia. Mild elevation in HbF can be seen. Microcytic polycythemia is a distinguishing feature that differentiates thalassemic disorders from iron deficiency, and thus the elevated RBC count in this case is more consistent with thalassemic disorder than iron deficiency.

QUESTION 2

Your patient recommends you to one of his relatives with a similar life-long history of anemia. Physical examination discloses splenomegaly. Evaluation of his relative reveals hemoglobin of 8.4 g/dL, RBC count of 4,900,000/μL, MCV of 65 fL, and platelet count of 361,000/μL. Peripheral blood smear is shown below. On methylene blue staining, RBC exhibited the appearance of golf balls.

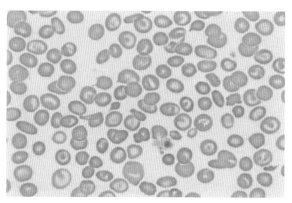

CASE FIGURE 10-2

✯ What is the most likely diagnosis?

A. HbH disease
B. Beta thalassemia major
C. Iron-deficiency anemia
D. Myelofibrosis
E. G6PD deficiency

Answer: A. HbH disease results from deletion of 3 alpha globin genes and presents as a more severe hypochromic microcytic anemia with underlying hemolysis and splenomegaly. Patients may require RBC transfusion support, and secondary iron overload is common. Peripheral blood staining with methylene blue reveals the typical golf ball appearance of RBC secondary to precipitated HbH.

A 74-year-old male with history of coronary and peripheral arterial disease presents to the emergency department complaining of a painful, blue, fourth right toe. Patient reports progressively worsening dark blue discoloration over the last 3 days. Patient also reports several months of burning sensation in his hands and feet and left upper quadrant discomfort. Laboratory workup reveals leukocyte count of 15,200/μL, hemoglobin of 14.6 g/dL, and platelet count of 825,000/μL. Peripheral blood smear and bone marrow aspirate are shown below.

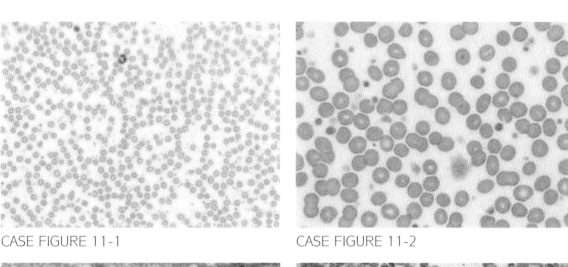

CASE FIGURE 11-1

CASE FIGURE 11-2

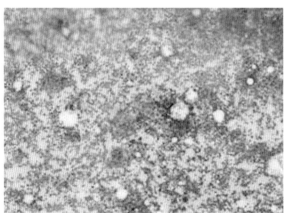

CASE FIGURE 11-3

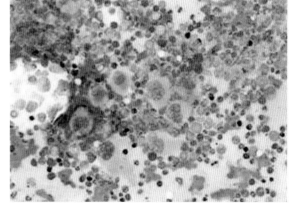

CASE FIGURE 11-4

QUESTION 1

⋆ What is the most likely diagnosis?

A. Reactive thrombocytosis

B. Iron deficiency

C. Essential thrombocytosis

Answer: C. Patient presents with elevated platelet and leukocyte counts and normal hemoglobin levels. Peripheral slide review reveals evidence of giant platelets with variable granulation. Bone marrow biopsy reveals megakaryocyte hyperplasia with clustering. This presentation is most consistent with essential thrombocytosis (ET). Iron-deficiency anemia and underlying conditions can be associated with secondary thrombocytosis; however, giant platelets with variable granules would not be expected. Clustering of megakaryocytes would also not be expected in secondary thrombocytosis. Normal hemoglobin level argues against underlying iron deficiency.

QUESTION 2

⋆ What would be the next most appropriate step in management?

A. Testing for BCR-ABL gene rearrangement

B. Testing for MPL mutation

C. Testing for JAK2 mutation

D. Both A and C

E. Testing for thrombopoietin level (TPO)

Answer: D. Mutations in JAK2 have been reported in approximately 40% to 50% of ET cases (*Blood.* 2005;106(6):2162, *NEJM.* 2005;352(17):1779). Ruling out chronic myeloid leukemia (CML) is essential, given the completely different approach to management. Mutations in MPL gene have been reported in less than 5% of ET cases (*Blood.* 2006;108(10):3472, *Blood.* 2008;112(1):141). Testing for TPO levels is not useful in differentiating primary from secondary forms of thrombocytosis (*Br J Haematol.* 1997;99(2):281).

QUESTION 3

✭ What would be the most appropriate management of this patient?

A. Aspirin

B. Hydroxyurea

C. Anagrelide

D. Aspirin and hydroxyurea

E. Aspirin and anagrelide

Answer: D. Patient falls into a high-risk category based on his age (greater than 60) and the presence of coronary and peripheral arterial disease. Thus, current evidence suggests that treatment with hydroxyurea and aspirin would constitute the most appropriate choice (*J Clin Oncol.* 2011;29(6):761).

CASE 12

A 31-year-old graduate student from Africa who immigrated to the Unites States 6 months previously presents to the emergency department complaining of generalized fatigue and dark urine for 1-week duration. Patient denies fever or recent infections. Physical examination reveals an alert and fully oriented female with pallor. Laboratory workup shows hemoglobin of 4.1 g/dL, mean corpuscular volume (MCV) of 106 fL, leukocyte count of 7,500/μL, platelet count of 34,000/μL, and LDH of 3,700 U/L. Urine is grossly dark, and analysis reveals 1–2 RBC/HPF. Direct antiglobin test is negative. Peripheral blood smear is shown below.

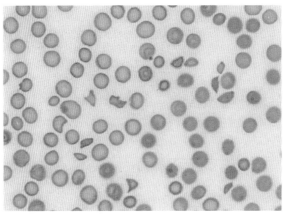

CASE FIGURE 12-1

QUESTION 1

★ What is the most likely diagnosis?

A. Hemoglobin H disease
B. Beta thalassemia major
C. Aplastic anemia (AA)
D. Thrombotic thrombocytopenic purpura (TTP)
E. Autoimmune hemolytic anemia (AIHA)

Answer: D. Peripheral slide reveals increased number of fragmented red blood cells (RBC)—schistocytes. This is characteristic of microangiopathic hemolytic anemia (MAHA). The clinical picture of MAHA, thrombocytopenia, negative direct antiglobin test, and hemoglobinuria (1–2 RBC/HPF in urine) supports the diagnosis of TTP.

QUESTION 2

✷ Plasma exchange was promptly initiated. Review of patient's medications reviewed no culprit agents. There was no evidence of underlying autoimmune disorder. Levels of ADAMTS13 returned at 23%. What would be an appropriate test to perform to elucidate the etiology of her presentation?

A. Complement level

B. Flow cytometry

C. HIV

D. IFN-gamma release assay

E. Bone marrow biopsy

Answer: C. HIV infection has been associated with TTP and HIV test was positive in the patient. The mechanism appears to be related to HIV-induced endothelial injury. Majority of HIV-associated TTP occurs in patients with advanced disease. Incidence appears to be lower in the HAART era, and initiation of HAART is considered essential in HIV-associated TTP (*Clin Infect Dis.* 2002;35(12):1534, *Clin Infect Dis.* 2004;39(suppl 5):S267, *Clin Infect Dis.* 2009;48(8):1129, *Kidney Int.* 2003;63(1):385, *Kidney Int.* 2003;63(5):1618, *Br J Haematol.* 2011;153(4):515).

A 65-year-old male presents for further evaluation secondary to progressive dyspnea on exertion, orthopnea, and left upper quadrant abdominal pain. Physical examination reveals massive splenomegaly and bilateral lower extremity edema. Laboratory workup shows hemoglobin of 9.3 g/dL, leukocyte count of 18,500/μL, and platelets of 458,000/μL. Peripheral blood smear is shown below.

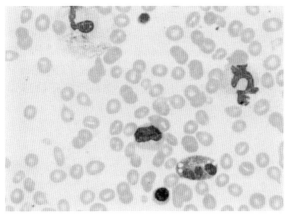

CASE FIGURE 13-1

QUESTION 1

✭ What is the most likely diagnosis?

A. Hemolytic anemia
B. Beta thalassemia major
C. Myelofibrosis
D. Myelodysplastic syndrome
E. Iron-deficiency anemia

Answer: C. Peripheral blood smear shows nucleated red blood cells (RBC), dacrocytes (teardrop RBCs), and giant platelets. This picture in concert with splenomegaly is most consistent with myelofibrosis. Myelodysplastic syndrome can also present with nucleated and teardrop RBCs in the peripheral blood; however, the elevated platelet and leukocyte count in addition to splenomegaly make this less likely. Bone marrow biopsy and reticulin staining of the bone marrow sample demonstrated extensive fibrosis.

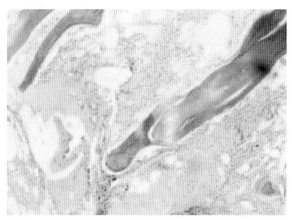

CASE FIGURE 13-2

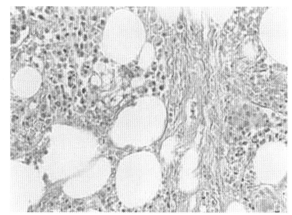

CASE FIGURE 13-3

QUESTION 2

⭐ What is the most appropriate next step in the management?

A. Testing for JAK2 mutation
B. Testing for MPL mutation
C. Testing for BCR-ABL translocation
D. Bone marrow biopsy
E. Both A and C

Answer: E. Mutations in JAK2 have been reported in approximately 50% of cases with myelofibrosis (*NEJM*. 2005;352(17):1779, *Blood*. 2005;106(6):2162). Mutations in MPL gene have been reported in 5% of cases with myelofibrosis regardless of JAK2 mutational status and in approximately 10% of cases with JAK2 negative myelofibrosis. Test for BCR-ABL is required to rule out CML (*Blood*. 2006;108(10):3472, *Br J Haematol*. 2010;149(2):250).

QUESTION 3

Chest x-ray was obtained secondary to orthopnea and lower extremity edema and is shown below.

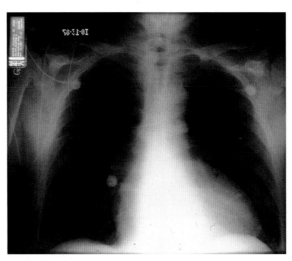

CASE FIGURE 13-4

✮ What is the most likely etiology of patient's complaints?

A. Congestive heart failure

B. Extramedullary hematopoiesis

C. Pulmonary embolism

D. Anemia

E. Hyperviscosity

Answer: B. Chest x-ray reveals enlarged globular cardiac silhouette with indistinct borders. This finding in the context of myelofibrosis is suggestive of involvement by extremedullary hematopoiesis. Pericardial biopsy revealed histologic findings of extramedullary hematopoiesis, and he was treated with low-dose radiation therapy. Involvement by extramedullary hematopoiesis in cases of myelofibrosis has been reported to affect any organ or organ system. Low-dose radiotherapy is considered the optimal palliative treatment for local foci of extremedullary hematopoiesis (*Mayo Clin Proc.* 2003; 78(10):1223).

A 28-year-old female with no significant prior medical history presents for further evaluation secondary to fatigue. Physical examination reveals pallor and splenomegaly. Laboratory workup shows leukocyte count of 76,000/μL, hemoglobin 8.5 g/dL, and platelet count of 34,000/μL. Peripheral blood slide is shown below.

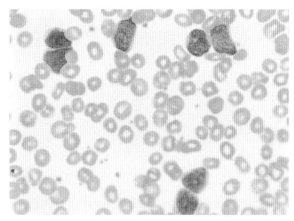

CASE FIGURE 14-1

Peripheral blood flow cytometry reveals increased number of leukocytes positive for TdT, CD10, and CD19.

QUESTION 1

☆ What is the most likely diagnosis?

A. Acute promyelocytic leukemia (APL)
B. Chronic myeloid leukemia (CML)
C. Chronic lymphocytic leukemia (CLL)
D. B-cell acute lymphoblastic leukemia (B-ALL)
E. T-cell acute lymphoblastic leukemia (T-ALL)

Answer: D. Peripheral blood smear reveals the presence of large cells with fine chromatin and increased nuclear-to-cytoplasmic ratio with a thin rim of cytoplasm. These findings are compatible with the description of blasts. Flow cytometry is positive for B-cell markers confirming the diagnosis of B-ALL.

QUESTION 2

✶ What is the most appropriate next test to perform in terms of patient's management and prognosis?

A. Bone marrow biopsy

B. HLA typing

C. Family history

D. Testing for BCR-ABL translocation

E. Lumbar puncture

Answer: D. All of the choices are reasonable; however, the single most important piece of information that will radically affect patient's management and prognosis is positivity for BCR-ABL transcript. Philadelphia positive ALL constitutes 20% to 30% of adult ALL cases and is a marker of high risk and poor prognosis. Incorporation of tyrosine kinase inhibitors into ALL treatment regimens is currently considered standard of care (*Blood.* 2010;115(2):206, *Blood.* 1999;93(11):3983, *Blood.* 1992;80(12):2983, *Blood.* 2007;109(4):1408, *J Clin Oncol.* 2010;28(22):3644, *Br J Haematol.* 2009;145(5):581).

CASE 15

A 43-year-old female with extensive history of alcohol use complicated by cirrhosis presents for evaluation secondary to progressively increasing ascites and fatigue. Evaluation reveals a jaundiced female with extensive ascites. Laboratory evaluation reveals hemoglobin of 6.4 g/dL, leukocyte count of 3,200/μL, and platelet count of 54,000/μL. Total bilirubin is elevated at 9.6 mg/dL, with an indirect component of 5.4 mg/dL. Peripheral blood smear is shown below.

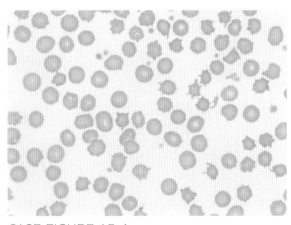

CASE FIGURE 15-1

QUESTION 1

☆ What is the most likely diagnosis?

A. Autoimmune hemolytic anemia

B. Hypersplenism

C. Alcohol-induced bone marrow suppression

D. Spur cell anemia

E. Thrombotic thrombocytopenic purpura

Answer: D. The peripheral blood smear reveals abnormal red blood cells with irregular and asymmetric protrusions with knobby ends of different sizes called acanthocytes (spur cells). In addition to liver disease, acanthocytes can be seen in abetalipoproteinemia, McLeod syndrome, neuroacanthocytosis syndromes, anorexia nervosa, myelodysplastic syndrome, and postsplenectomy. Spur cell anemia presents as a hemolytic anemia seen in cases of advanced liver disease, especially alcoholic liver disease and alcoholic cirrhosis. Echinocytes (burr cells), on the other hand, are red blood cells with regular and symmetrical short protrusions of similar sizes. Echinocytes are most commonly artifactual, but can also be seen in severe renal disease. Peripheral blood smears contrasting acanthocytes with echinocytes are shown below (*Hepatol Res.* 2010;40(2):161).

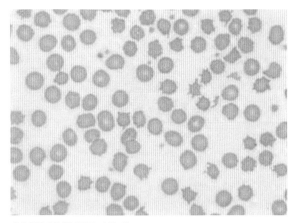

CASE FIGURE 15-2

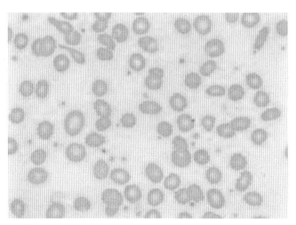

CASE FIGURE 15-3

CASE 16

A 49-year-old male presented for further evaluation secondary to weakness and fatigue. Physical examination revealed splenomegaly with no peripheral lymphadenopathy. Laboratory workup showed leukocyte count of 18,500/μL, hemoglobin of 9.3 g/dL, and platelet count of 110,000/μL. Peripheral blood smear is shown below.

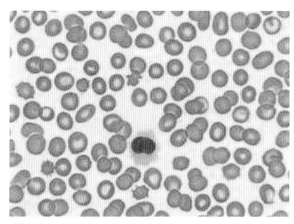

CASE FIGURE 16-1

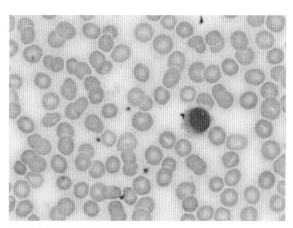

CASE FIGURE 16-2

QUESTION 1

★ What is the most likely diagnosis?

A. Chronic lymphocytic leukemia (CLL)

B. Chronic myeloid leukemia (CML)

C. Hairy cell leukemia (HCL)

D. Large granular lymphocyte leukemia (LGL)

E. Prolymphocytic leukemia (PLL)

Answer: C. Peripheral blood smear reveals the presence of lymphocytes with abnormal "hairy" cytoplasmic projections, which in the context of splenomegaly and absent peripheral lymphadenopathy are highly suggestive of HCL. Hairy cell leukemia is a rare indolent lymphoproliferative disorder that occurs primarily in males. Patients typically present with weakness, fatigue, and left upper quadrant pain due to splenomegaly. Monocytopenia is a characteristic finding in the peripheral blood.

QUESTION 2

✫ What is the typical flow cytometry pattern seen in cases of HCL?

A. CD11c+, CD20+, CD23−, CD25+, CD103+, CD123+, cyclin D1+

B. CD5+, CD20+, CD23+, CD25+, CD103−, CD123−, cyclin D1+

C. CD11c−, CD20+, CD23+, CD25+, CD103+, CD123+, cyclin D1+

D. CD11c−, CD20+, CD23−, CD25+, CD103+, CD123+, cyclin D1−

E. CD11c−, CD20+, CD23−, CD25+, CD103+, CD123+, cyclin D1+

Answer: A. Positivity for common B-cell markers, CD11c, CD25, CD103, CD123, and cyclin D1 are characteristic for HCL. Expression of CD23 is typically negative (*Blood*. 1993;82(4):1277).

QUESTION 3

✫ What genetic test can be used to confirm the diagnosis?

A. Testing for KIT mutations

B. Testing for RAS mutations

C. Testing for EGFR mutations

D. Testing for ALK mutations

E. Testing for BRAF mutations

Answer: E. Mutations in BRAF have been detected in nearly 100% of HCL cases and can be used as a diagnostic test to differentiate HCL from other lymphoproliferative disorders (*NEJM*. 2011; 364(24):2305, *Br J Haematol*. 2011;155(5):609, *Blood*. 2012;119(1):188, *Blood*. 2012;119(1):192).

A 67-year-old male is referred by his primary care physician for further evaluation of elevated hemoglobin level. Patient reports feeling generally well; however, on review of systems, he does report mild fatigue and left abdominal discomfort. Patient is a non-smoker with no history of cardiac or pulmonary disease. Examination reveals a male with a ruddy complexion and splenomegaly. Laboratory workup shows hemoglobin of 19.5 g/dL, mean corpuscular volume 79 fL, leukocyte count of 19,800/μL, and platelet count of 356,000/μL. Peripheral blood smear shows no gross abnormalities. Testing for JAK2 V617F mutation is instead of returned positive, and patient is diagnosed with polycythemia vera (PV).

QUESTION 1

Patient is treated appropriately and is followed for the next 9 years until he notes progressive increase in his abdominal girth and fatigue. Physical examination reveals increased splenomegaly. Hemoglobin level is found to be 8.7 g/dL, leukocyte count 9,800/μL, and platelets count 115,000/μL. Peripheral blood smear is shown below.

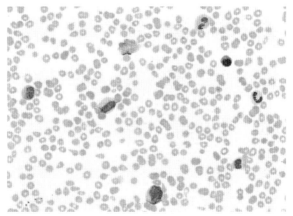

CASE FIGURE 17-1

* What is the most likely explanation of patient's presentation?

A. Splenic vein thrombosis

B. Budd Chiari syndrome

C. Transformation to acute leukemia

D. Transformation to myelofibrosis

E. Chronic gastrointestinal bleeding

Answer: D. Peripheral blood smear reveals abnormal teardrop-shaped red blood cells, nucleated red blood cells, and promyelocytes. There is no evidence of blasts. This picture is most consistent with progression to post-PV myelofibrosis. Progression to post-PV myelofibrosis has been reported with a frequency of 16% at 10 years and 34% at 15 years of follow-up (*Br J Haematol.* 2009;146(5):504).

QUESTION 2

After a period of 3 more years, the patient presents to the emergency department complaining of fatigue and dyspnea on exertion. Physical examination reveals petechiae on both lower extremities. Laboratory evaluation reveals a hemoglobin of 7.6 g/dL, leukocyte count of 36,200/μL, and platelet count of 22,000/μL. Peripheral blood smear is shown below.

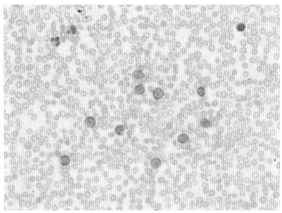

CASE FIGURE 17-2   CASE FIGURE 17-3

* What is the most likely diagnosis?

A. Progression to acute leukemia

B. Aplastic anemia

C. Transformation to chronic myeloid leukemia

D. Immune thrombocytopenic purpura

E. Autoimmune hemolytic anemia

Answer: A. Peripheral blood smear reveals large leukocytes with high nuclear-to-cytoplasmic ratio with fine chromatin consistent with blasts. Flow cytometry was positive for CD13 and CD33 while myeloperoxidase stain was positive confirming the diagnosis of acute myeloid leukemia. Transformation to acute leukemia has been reported in less than 5% of cases of post-PV or primary myelofibrosis (*Blood.* 2005;105(3):973, *Blood.* 2005;105(7):2664).

CASE 18

A 47-year-old male presents for further evaluation secondary to worsening fatigue of 2 weeks' duration. Laboratory evaluation reveals elevated leukocyte count at 47,000/μL, hemoglobin of 10.3 g/dL, platelet count of 67,000/μL, and LDH of 2,300/μL. Peripheral blood smear is obtained and is shown below.

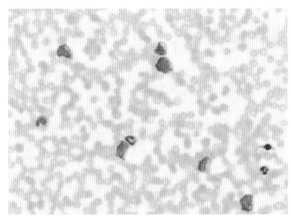

CASE FIGURE 18-1

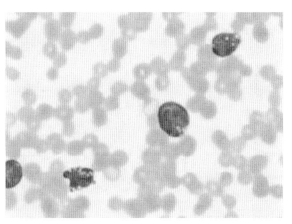

CASE FIGURE 18-2

Patient is admitted to the hospital, and bone marrow aspiration is obtained as shown below.

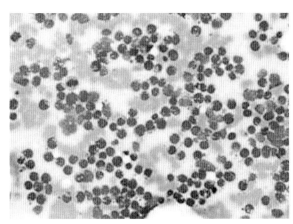

CASE FIGURE 18-3

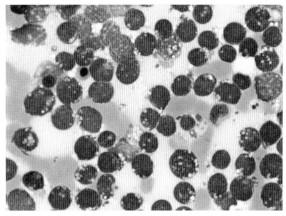

CASE FIGURE 18-4

Flow cytometry revealed an increased population of cells bearing CD10, CD19, CD20, CD79a with negative expression of CD5, terminal deoxytransferase (TdT), myeloperoxidase (MPO), and cyclin D1.

QUESTION 1

✯ What is the most likely diagnosis?

A. Acute monoblastic leukemia (AML)

B. Chronic myeloid leukemia (CML)

C. Mantle cell lymphoma in leukemic phase (MCL)

D. Acute lymphoblastic leukemia (ALL)

E. Burkitt lymphoma/leukemia (BL)

Answer: E. Peripheral slide reveals increased number of leukocytes exhibiting high nuclear-to-cytoplasmic ratio with basophilic cytoplasm and prominent vacuoles in the cytoplasm and overlying the nucleus. These are the typical features of Burkitt lymphoma/leukemia. Negativity for MPO and the presence of B-cell markers on flow cytometry rules out AML. Negativity for TdT differentiates BL from ALL that is virtually always positive for TdT.

QUESTION 2

✯ What is the most common chromosomal abnormality in Burkitt lymphoma/leukemia?

A. t(11;14)

B. t(2;8)

C. t(14;18)

D. t(8;14)

E. t(8;22)

Answer: D. t(8;14) involving the immunoglobulin heavy chain on chromosome 14 has been reported in 80% of BL cases and leads to overexpression of the oncogene *c-MYC*. Translocations involving kappa and lambda light chains on chromosomes 2 and 22, respectively, are seen in 15% and 5% of cases (*J Clin Oncol.* 2000;18(21):3707, *Proc Natl Acad Sci USA.* 1982;79(24):7824).

A 79-year-old male with no significant prior medical history presents for further evaluation of fatigue and generalized weakness for the last several months. He denies night sweats and fever. Physical examination shows no splenomegaly or lymphadenopathy. Laboratory evaluation discloses hemoglobin of 10.1 g/dL, MCV of 110 fL, leukocyte count of 5,600/μL, and platelet count of 136,000/μL. Peripheral blood smear is shown below.

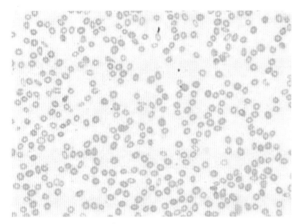

CASE FIGURE 19-1

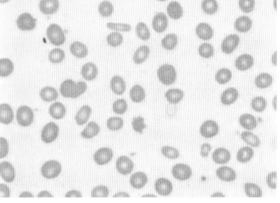

CASE FIGURE 19-2

Vitamin B$_{12}$ and folate levels are normal. Patient denied alcohol use. Bone marrow biopsy is obtained and shows a hypercellular bone marrow. Sample of bone marrow aspirate in addition to a Prussian blue–stained specimen are shown below.

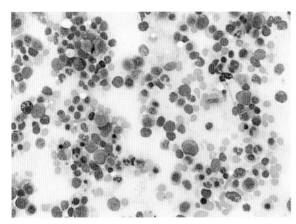

CASE FIGURE 19-3

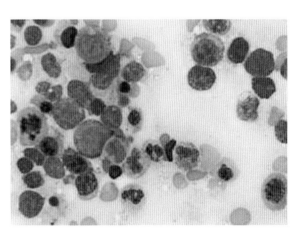

CASE FIGURE 19-4

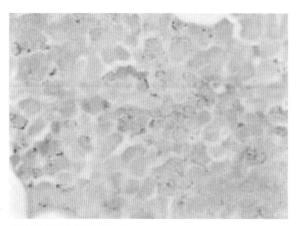

CASE FIGURE 19-5

QUESTION 1

✩ What is the most likely diagnosis?

A. Refractory anemia with ring sideroblasts (RARS)

B. Autoimmune hemolytic anemia (AIHA)

C. Immune thrombocytopenic purpura (ITP)

D. Acute myeloid leukemia (AML)

E. Myelofibrosis (MF)

Answer: A. Peripheral blood smear exhibits red blood cells (RBC) of different morphologies with ovalocytes, teardrop-shaped RBCs, and few acanthocytes. There also appears to be at least two different red blood cell populations, one that is more normal appearing and the other with hypochromia and anisopoikilocytosis. Bone marrow sample reveals evidence of dysplastic erythropoiesis, nuclear budding and cytoplastic vacuoles in RBC precursors, defective granulation of myeloid progenitors, and increased ring sideroblasts. There is no evidence of bone marrow fibrosis. This clinical presentation is most consistent with RARS. It has been recently reported that SF3B1 haploinsufficiency leads to ring sideroblast formation in patients with myelodysplastic syndromes (*Blood.* 2012;120:73–3186, *Blood.* 1982;59(2):293).

CASE 20

A 57-year-old male truck driver presents for evaluation of chest pain and dyspnea on minimal exertion. Patient reports gradually worsening generalized fatigue over the preceding 3 months. Examination reveals splenomegaly. Laboratory workup shows leukocyte count of 32,000/μL, hemoglobin of 9.7 g/dL, and platelet count of 134,000/μL. Peripheral blood smear reveals increased number of homogeneously appearing leukocytes as shown below.

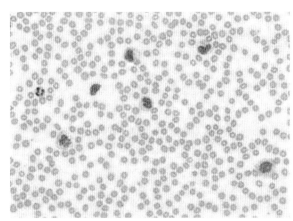

CASE FIGURE 20-1   CASE FIGURE 20-2

QUESTION 1

★ What is the next most appropriate test to perform?

A. Leukocyte alkaline phosphatase

B. BCR-ABL translocation

C. Flow cytometry

D. CT chest/abdomen/pelvis

E. Spleen biopsy

Answer: B. Peripheral blood count reveals increased number of monocytes. The clinical picture of increased leukocyte count, absolute monocytosis, and splenomegaly raise concern for underlying chronic myeloid leukemia (CML) or chronic myelomonocytic leukemia (CMML). Testing for BCR-ABL translocation will differentiate between the two as CML is by definition positive while CMML is negative for BCR-ABL translocation (*Leukemia.* 2008;22(7):1308).

QUESTION 2

Testing for BCl-ABL translocation is negative, and a bone marrow aspirate is hypercellular and shows 2% myeloblasts. A diagnosis of CMML is made, and the patient is treated with oral etoposide for the next 18 months with near normalization of his peripheral blood counts and decreased splenomegaly. On a routine follow-up, the patient is noted to have increased leukocyte count of 45,800/μL, hemoglobin of 8.2 g/dL, and platelet count of 24,000/μL. Peripheral blood smear is shown below.

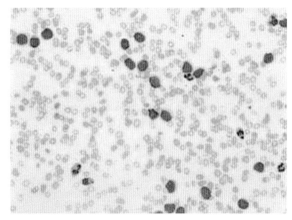

CASE FIGURE 20-3

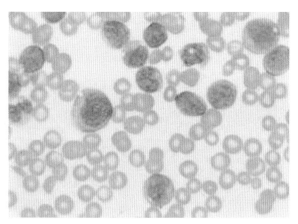

CASE FIGURE 20-4

✯ What is the most likely explanation of the new clinical picture?

A. Progression to myelofibrosis (MF)

B. Etoposide-induced toxicity

C. Progression to acute myelomonocytic leukemia (AMML)

D. De novo acute lymphoblastic leukemia (ALL)

E. Transformation to chronic myeloid leukemia (CML)

Answer: C. Peripheral blood smear now exhibits a different picture compared with the one observed at diagnosis with predominance of monocytoid cells with increased nuclear-to-cytoplasmic ratio and fine chromatin and nucleoli. This picture is consistent with transformation to AMML. CMML is a myeloproliferative/myelodysplastic syndrome with a variable survival. Two large case series of CMML reported a median survival of 12 and 18 months respectively. The most important factor determining survival is the percentage of blasts in the bone marrow and blood, with transformation to acute leukemia reported in approximately 20% to 40% of patients.

A 56-year-old female presents for evaluation of malaise and a recent unintentional 10-pound weight loss. Patient reports no night sweats or fevers, but reports enlarged lymph nodes in her neck area. She also mentions several weeks of epistaxis and blurry vision. Physical examination confirms cervical lymphadenopathy and splenomegaly, and petechiae involving both lower extremities. Fundoscopic exam shows retinal hemorrhages and engorged retinal veins. Laboratory evaluation shows leukocytes of 12,700/μL, hemoglobin of 10.8 g/dL, and platelet count of 178,000/μL. Peripheral slide is shown below.

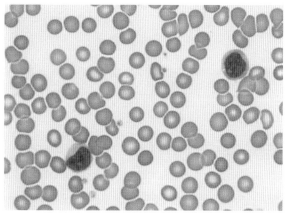

CASE FIGURE 21-1

Bone marrow biopsy is obtained and shows a hypercellular bone marrow with diffuse involvement by small lymphocytes as shown below. Flow cytometry revealed positivity for CD19, CD20, and CD138, with negative expression of CD5 and CD23.

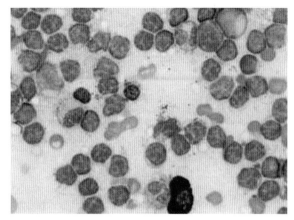

CASE FIGURE 21-2

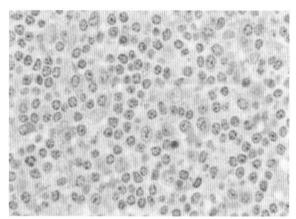

CASE FIGURE 21-3

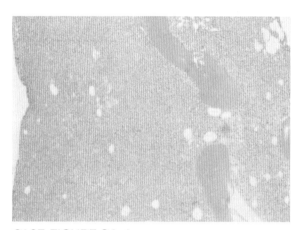

CASE FIGURE 21-4

QUESTION 1

☆ What is the most likely diagnosis?

A. Follicular lymphoma (FL)

B. Small lymphocytic lymphoma/chronic lymphocytic leukemia (SLL/CLL)

C. Lymphoplasmacytic lymphoma (LPL)

D. Mantle cell lymphoma (MCL)

E. Diffuse large B-cell lymphoma (DLBCL)

Answer: C. Peripheral smear reveals the presence of circulating cells with plasmacytoid features. These cells resemble lymphocytes and are characterized by the presence of basophilic cytoplasm, eccentric nucleus with perinuclear clearing, similar to plasma cells. Chromatin can be found in a typical clock-face pattern as seen above. The bone marrow is typically diffusely infiltrated by the LPL cells, and mast cells can also be seen (deeply basophilic cell above). LPL is an indolent small B-cell lymphoma, and the peripheral blood shows a leukemic phase in approximately 30% of cases. Waldenstrom macroglobulinemia (WM) is a specific subtype of LPL and is defined as LPL with bone marrow involvement associated with IgM monoclonal gammopathy and may present with symptoms related to hyperviscosity. Expression of typical plasma cell markers (CD138) supports the diagnosis of LPL/WM. Lack of CD5 and CD23 expression makes the diagnosis of SLL/CLL and MCL less likely (*Br J Haematol.* 2001;115(3):575, *Semin Oncol.* 2003;30(2):110, *J Clin Oncol.* 2005;23(7):1564).

QUESTION 2

✯ What is the most common structural chromosomal abnormality seen in cases of LPL?

A. t(9;14)

B. t(9;11)

C. t(14;18)

D. del(5q)

E. del(6q)

Answer: E. Chromosomal abnormalities are seen in 32% of LPL cases, and approximately 50% of LPL cases with chromosomal abnormalities exhibit del(6q). Recent studies have shown that the previously reported t(9;14) is less common than originally described and is currently considered a rare feature (*Am J Clin Pathol.* 2001;116(4):543, *Hum Pathol.* 2004;35(4):447, *Adv Anat Pathol.* 2005;12(5):246).

A 31-year-old African American female is admitted to the hospital with diffuse lower back in addition to right shoulder and knee pain. Patient reports several similar episodes previously. Physical examination reveals decreased range of motion in affected joints secondary to pain with no obvious swelling. Laboratory evaluation reveals hemoglobin of 7.7 g/dL, mean corpuscular volume (MCV) of 85 fL, and normal leukocyte and platelet counts. Peripheral smear is shown below.

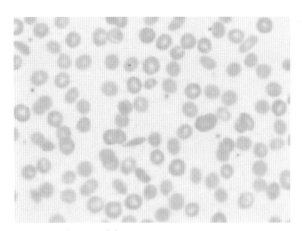 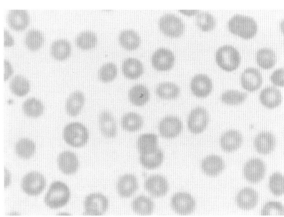

CASE FIGURE 22-1   CASE FIGURE 22-2

QUESTION 1

⭐ What is the most likely underlying condition?

A. Beta thalassemia major

B. Hemoglobin H disease

C. Sickle-beta thalassemia

D. Sickle cell trait

E. Sickle cell disease

Answer: E. The case describes a young African American female with multifocal bone pain. Laboratory evaluation reveals a moderately severe normocytic anemia. Normal MCV argues strongly against thalassemia. Peripheral blood smear reveals few sickled red blood cells (RBC) in addition to few basophilic RBC inclusions representing Howell–Jolly bodies, which are nuclear remnants that are removed by the spleen. Their presence in the peripheral blood is suggestive of decreased splenic function. Functional asplenia is an early complication of sickle cell disease that is evident within the first year of life. Nuclear medicine spleen and liver scan was obtained and revealed nearly absent splenic uptake consistent with functional asplenia (*Blood.* 2011;117(9):2614, *Lancet.* 2011;378(9785):86).

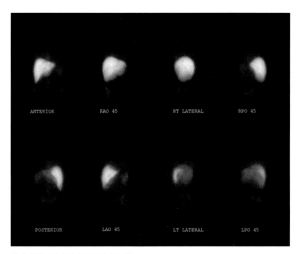

CASE FIGURE 22-3

CASE 23

A 62-year-old male presents for evaluation of bilateral cervical, axillary, and inguinal lymphadenopathy. Physical examination confirms these findings in addition to disclosing splenomegaly. Laboratory evaluation reveals leukocyte count of 70,000/μL, hemoglobin of 9.6 g/dL, and platelet count of 138,000/μL. Flow cytometry reveals increased population of cells expressing CD5, CD19, CD20, and CD23. Peripheral blood smear is shown below.

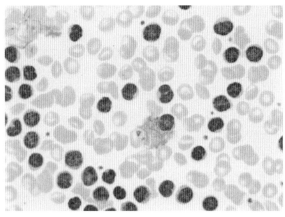

CASE FIGURE 23-1

QUESTION 1

⭐ What is the most likely diagnosis?

A. Mantle cell lymphoma (MCL)

B. Chronic lymphocytic leukemia (CLL)

C. Follicular lymphoma (FL)

D. Chronic myeloid leukemia (CML)

E. Acute lymphoblastic leukemia (ALL)

Answer: B. The presence of an increased number of mature-appearing lymphocytes with small amount of cytoplasm and clumped chromatin, in addition to flow cytometry revealing increased expression of CD5, CD20, and CD23 is characteristic of CLL. Positivity for CD23 differentiates CLL from MCL.

QUESTION 2

Patient was treated with 6 cycles of bendamustine and rituximab with normalization of peripheral blood counts and disappearance of lymphadenopathy. Over the next 3 years, the patient was followed with no evidence of active disease. However, during the fourth year of follow-up, he presented with multiple new skin lesions and fever. Laboratory findings revealed leukocyte count of 27,000/μL, hemoglobin of 11.9 g/dL, platelet count of 124,000/μL, and LDH of 547 U/L. Peripheral blood smear is shown.

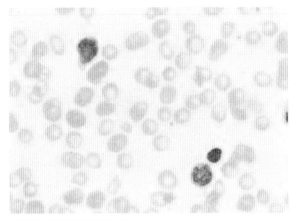

CASE FIGURE 23-2

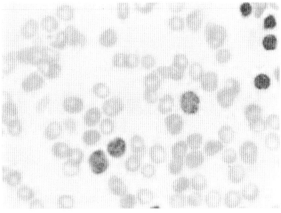

CASE FIGURE 23-3

☆ What is the most likely explanation of his presentation?

A. Transformation to prolymphocytic leukemia (PLL)

B. Transformation to aggressive lymphoma

C. Transformation to acute lymphoblastic leukemia (ALL)

D. Therapy-related myelodysplastic syndrome (t-MDS)

E. Relapse of chronic lymphocytic leukemia (CLL)

Answer: B. Peripheral blood slide reveals a different cell population from that observed originally at diagnosis. The abnormal cells are large with sparse cytoplasm, fine uncondensed chromatin, and no nucleoli. These cells do not resemble prolymphocytes that are characterized by their large size, some degree of chromatin condensation, increased amount of cytoplasm, and prominent nucleolus. Taken together with new skin lesions, B symptoms, and elevated LDH, the presentation is most consistent with a transformation to an aggressive lymphoma, Richter's transformation (RT). Skin biopsy was obtained and histiologic exam revealed diffuse large B-cell lymphoma (DLBCL). DLBCL is the most common histology seen in RT; however, rare cases of Hodgkin lymphoma and even T-cell lymphomas have been reported. Below is a comparison between the peripheral blood picture in RT and PLL (*Cancer*. 2005;103(2):216, *Br J Haematol*. 2012;156(1):50, *Am J Clin Pathol*. 1990;93(3):333, *Am J Clin Pathol*. 1995;103(3):348).

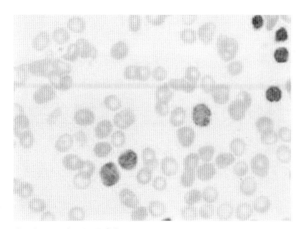
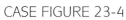

CASE FIGURE 23-4

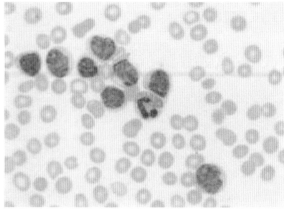

CASE FIGURE 23-5

A 86-year-old female is referred for evaluation of fatigue. Physical examination reveals no lymphadenopathy or hepatosplenomegaly. Laboratory workup shows a leukocyte count of 3,100/μL, hemoglobin of 8.1 g/dL, mean corpuscular volume of 89 fL, reticulocyte count of 2.4%, and platelet count of 32,000/μL. Peripheral blood smear is shown below.

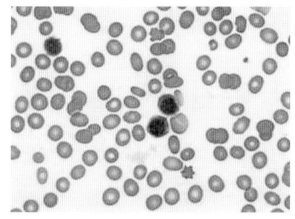

CASE FIGURE 24-1

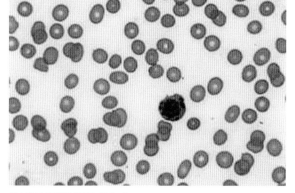

CASE FIGURE 24-2

Bone marrow aspiration is obtained and is shown below.

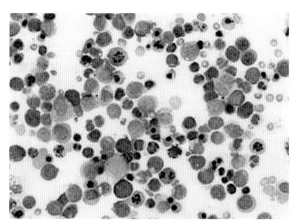

CASE FIGURE 24-3

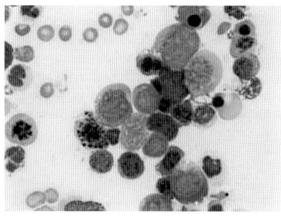

CASE FIGURE 24-4

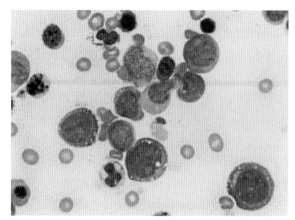

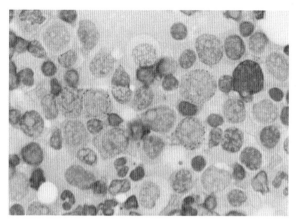

CASE FIGURE 24-5   CASE FIGURE 24-6

Flow cytometry revealed lack of CD13, CD33, CD34, and HLA-DR expression. Myeloperoxidase (MPO) testing returned negative while glycophorin was positive.

QUESTION 1

☆ What is the most likely diagnosis?

A. Acute megakaryoblastic leukemia

B. Acute promyelocytic leukemia

C. Acute erythroid leukemia

D. Burkitt lymphoma in leukemia phase

E. Myelofibrosis

Answer: C. Peripheral blood smear exhibits the presence of abnormal cells resembling erythroid precursors, with nuclear irregularity and fragmentation. Bone marrow aspirate shows increased number of erythroid precursors exhibiting gigantism, karyorrhexis, multinucleation, and cytoplasmic and perinuclear vacuoles that are periodic-acid Schiff positive (Fig. 24-6), findings that are characteristic of acute erythroid leukemia (Di Guglielmo disease). Erythroblasts do not express myeloid lineage markers and do not stain for MPO. Positivity for glycophorin, a red blood cell membrane glycoprotein, and reaction with antihemoglobin antibodies can provide diagnostic clues. Cytoplasmic vacuoles are also seen in Burkitt lymphoma/leukemia and can result in diagnostic confusion, but the vacuoles in BL stain positive with Oil-red-O for lipid (*Blood*. 2010;115(10):1985).

CASE 25

A 58-year-old female presents for further evaluation of left shoulder and back pain. Patient reports several month history of intermittent skin rash and itching. Physical examination reveals mild splenomegaly. Laboratory workup shows hemoglobin of 12.3 g/dL, leukocyte count of 7,600/μL, and platelet count of 198,000/μL. Imaging of her left shoulder and spine notes several lytic lesions in the head of the humerus and diffuse osteopenia with several vertebral compression fractures. Bone marrow biopsy is obtained and is shown below.

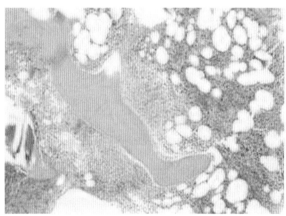

CASE FIGURE 25-1   CASE FIGURE 25-2

Serum tryptase levels are found to be elevated. Staining for CD25 and CD117 are positive.

QUESTION 1

⭐ What is the most likely diagnosis?

A. Systemic mastocytosis
B. Metastatic malignancy
C. Acute myeloid leukemia with eosinophilia
D. Chronic myeloid leukemia
E. Myelofibrosis

Answer: A. Bone marrow biopsy reveals a paratrabecular infiltrate by spindle-shaped hypergranular cells with irregular nuclei. Clusters of eosinophils are concentrated at the periphery of the infiltrate. Positivity for CD25 and CD117 in addition to elevated tryptase levels is characteristic of mastocytosis. Diffuse musculoskeletal pain, osteopenia, and osteoporosis are associated with systemic mastocytosis. Serum tryptase level and staining for tryptase are useful diagnostic tools. Mutations in KIT (CD117) are detected in more than 90% of cases, and D816V mutation in KIT is the most common. Imatinib does not have clinical activity against D816V mutant KIT (*J Bone Miner Res.* 1990;5(8):871, *J Spinal Disord.* 1991;4(3):369, *Bone.* 2002;31(5):556, *NEJM.* 1987;316(26):1622, *Hematol Oncol Clin North Am.* 2000;14(3):641, *Blood.* 2006;108(7):2366, *Leuk Res.* 2009;33(11):1481, *J Mol Diagn.* 2006;8(4):412, *J Allergy Clin Immunol.* 2004;114(1):3, *Proc Natl Acad Sci USA.* 1995;92(23):10560).

CASE 26

A 37-year-old male with history of HIV with poor compliance with HAART presents for evaluation of 1 month of fever, fatigue, and weight loss. Review of systems does not point to a specific source of infectious process. Physical examination reveals splenomegaly. Laboratory workup shows hemoglobin of 9.2 g/dL, leukocyte count of 4,700/μL, and platelet count of 134,000/μL. The most recent CD4 cell count is 135/μL. Peripheral blood is shown below.

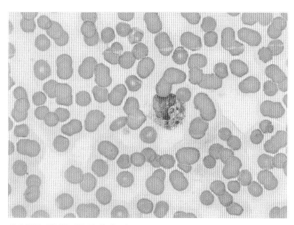

CASE FIGURE 26-1

Bone marrow aspirate is obtained and is shown below in addition to a silver-stained section of the bone marrow aspirate.

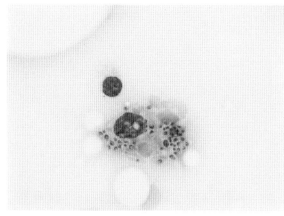

CASE FIGURE 26-2

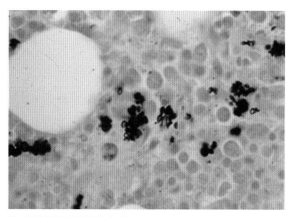

CASE FIGURE 26-3

QUESTION 1

✭ What is the most likely diagnosis?

A. Disseminated tuberculosis

B. Disseminated histoplasmosis

C. Disseminated mycobacterium avium complex infection

D. AIDS-related lymphoma

E. Hemophagocytosis

Answer: **B.** Peripheral blood smear and bone marrow demonstrate multiple intracellular crescent-ring organisms that stain positively with Gomori methamine silver (GMS) stain. This is a classical presentation of disseminated histoplasmosis associated with HIV infection. Blood and bone marrow cultures yielded Histoplasma capsulatum. Fever and weight loss are the most common manifestation of histoplasmosis and HIV infection. Anemia, neutropenia, or thrombocytopenia reflecting bone marrow involvement may be present. Between 5% and 10% of patients present with an acute illness with hypotension, disseminated intravascular coagulation, and shock. Careful inspection of the peripheral blood smear may be helpful in the evaluation of HIV patients with fever and anemia.

A 22-year-old HIV-positive male presents for further workup of fevers, fatigue, and weight loss. Patient reports that he underwent an extensive workup with no underlying etiology determined. Physical examination reveals bilateral cervical and axillary lymphadenopathy and no hepatosplenomegaly. Laboratory evaluation reveals hemoglobin of 8.1 g/dL, leukocyte count of 12,800/μL, and platelet count of 105,000/μL. Most recent CD4 cell count is 35/μL. Secondary to the presence of nucleated red blood cells in the peripheral blood, a bone marrow aspirate and biopsy was obtained. Peripheral blood and bone marrow samples are shown below.

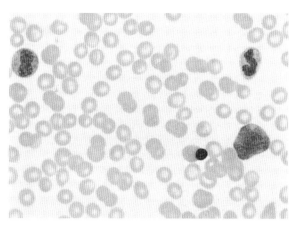

CASE FIGURE 27-1

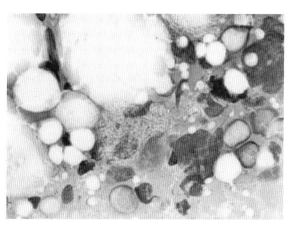

CASE FIGURE 27-2

QUESTION 1

★ What is the most appropriate step in the workup of this patient?

A. Testing bone marrow for the presence of lymphoma
B. Testing bone marrow for mycobacterium avium complex (MAC) infections
C. Flow cytometry of bone marrow aspirate
D. Check ferritin level
E. Check vitamin B$_{12}$ level

Answer: B. Blood smear shows leukoerythroblastosis, and a foamy macrophage "pseudo-Gaucher" cell is seen in the bone marrow aspirate (noted in above image); acid-fast stain (AFB) of the bone marrow aspirate revealed extensive involvement by mycobacteria (as seen below) that on further testing was found to represent MAC. MAC is usually a late clinical syndrome in HIV patients with CD4 counts less than 50. Weight loss, fatigue, fever, and anemia are common presenting manifestations in such patients. Several studies examined the clinical benefit and additional yield provided by bone marrow cultures or AFB stains compared with blood cultures alone. One retrospective study showed earlier positivity for bone marrow cultures compared with blood (22 vs. 24 days). Another study revealed that blood cultures and blood AFB staining were the most sensitive and quickest method to diagnose disseminated MAC as compared with bone marrow cultures and bone marrow AFB staining (*Am J Med.* 1998;104(2):123, *Am J Clin Pathol.* 1998;110(6):806, *Int J STD AIDS.* 2005;16(10):686).

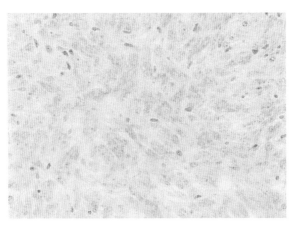

CASE FIGURE 27-3

A 78-year-old female presents for further evaluation of anemia. Physical examination reveals no lymphadenopathy or organomegaly. Laboratory evaluation shows hemoglobin of 8.2 g/dL, mean corpuscular volume of 106 fL, leukocyte count of 6,700/μL, and platelet count of 562,000/μL. Peripheral smear is shown below.

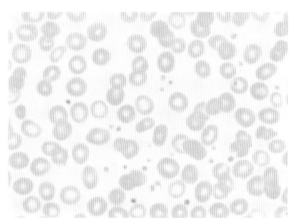

CASE FIGURE 28-1

Bone marrow aspiration and biopsy were obtained and revealed hypercellularity and no increased ring sideroblasts. Bone marrow aspirate is shown below.

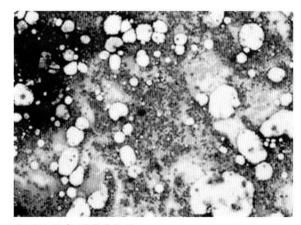

CASE FIGURE 28-2

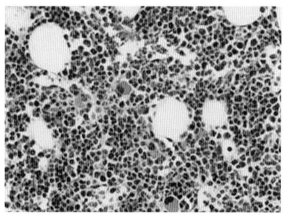

CASE FIGURE 28-3

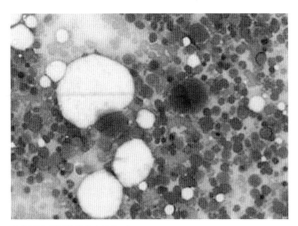

CASE FIGURE 28-4

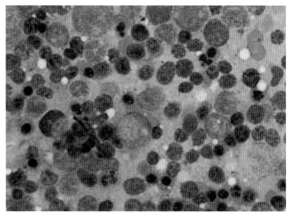

CASE FIGURE 28-5

QUESTION 1

✳ What is the most likely diagnosis?

A. Myeloproliferative neoplasm

B. Refractory anemia with ring sideroblasts with thrombocytosis (RARS-T)

C. Iron-deficiency anemia

D. 5q- syndrome

E. Vitamin B_{12} deficiency

Answer: D. The clinical case describes an elderly female presenting with moderate macrocytic anemia, thrombocytosis, and preserved leukocyte counts. Peripheral blood smear reveals evidence of anisopoikilocytosis. As demonstrated in the images of the bone marrow aspirate and biopsy, there is erythroid lineage dysplasia with nuclear budding and the characteristic hypolobated micromegakaryocytes characteristic of 5q- syndrome. This syndrome classically presents with female predominance, macrocytic anemia, thrombocytosis, preserved neutrophil count, increased number of hypolobated micromegakaryocytes, and low risk of progression to acute leukemia (*Leukemia*. 2010;24(7):1283).

QUESTION 2

✳ What is the most appropriate management of this patient?

A. Reduced intensity allogeneic hematopoietic stem cell transplantation

B. Hypomethylating agent (azacitidine or decitabine)

C. Cytarabine and daunorubicin (7 + 3 regimen)

D. Observation

E. Lenalidomide

Answer: E. Lenalidomide has shown remarkable activity in MDS with 5q- syndrome. Several studies documented transfusion independence and cytogenetic responses rate of 67% and 77%, respectively.

Studies have linked deletions in 5q to decreased expression of the ribosomal gene RPS14, whose product is required for the maturation of 40S ribosomal subunit. Additional studies have implicated decreased levels of micro-RNAs, miR-145 and miR-146a, that are encoded in proximity to RPS14 gene, in cases of 5q- syndrome (*Blood.* 2009;113(17):3947, *Br J Haematol.* 2008;140(3):267, *NEJM.* 2006;355(14):1456, *Blood.* 2011;118(14):3765, *Nature.* 2008;451(7176):335, *Br J Haematol.* 2008; 142(1)57, *Br J Haematol.* 2007;139(4):578, *Nat Med.* 2010;16(1):49).

CASE 29

A 62-year-old female with a history of discoid lupus presents complaining of fatigue. Physical examination reveals pallor and tachycardia. There is no evidence of lymphade-nopathy or hepatosplenomegaly. Laboratory workup reveals hemoglobin of 6.2 g/dL, mean corpuscular volume (MCV) of 122 fL, leukocyte count of 16,800/μL, and platelet count of 380,000/μL. Peripheral smear is shown below.

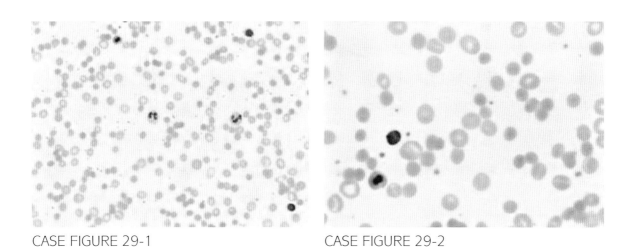

CASE FIGURE 29-1   CASE FIGURE 29-2

QUESTION 1

✷ What is the most likely etiology for the elevated MCV?

A. Vitamin B$_{12}$ deficiency

B. Folete deficiency

C. Reticulocytosis

D. Myelodysplastic syndrome

E. Hypothyroidism

Answer: C. Peripheral blood smear reveals increased number of large red blood cells (RBC) with basophilic staining (polychromasia), characteristic of reticulocytes. Given that reticulocytes have higher MCV values than mature RBCs (103-126 fL), the most likely etiology underlying the elevated MCV is reticulocytosis.

QUESTION 2

✮ What is the most likely diagnosis?

A. Iron-deficiency anemia

B. Anemia of chronic disease

C. Vitamin B_{12} deficiency

D. Folate deficiency

E. Hemolytic anemia

Answer: E. The constellation of symptoms is most consistent with hemolytic anemia. Further workup revealed reticulocyte percentage of 23.9%, direct antiglobin test being positive for IgG, and LDH being elevated at 675 U/L. Patient's presentation is consistent with autoimmune hemolytic anemia (AIHA) probably related to underlying discoid lupus. Corticosteroids are considered the first-line treatment option. Relapse of refractory AIHA can be treated with immunosuppression, rituximab, or splenectomy. The use of intravenous gamma globulins (IVIG) is considered a temporizing measure pending response to a more definitive treatment (*Am J Hematol.* 1993;44(4):237, *Blood.* 2010; 116(11):1831, *Semin Hematol.* 2005;42(3):131).

CASE 30

A 56-year-old female presents for evaluation of pancytopenia after presenting to her primary care physician, complaining of 3 months of fatigue and bleeding gums. Patient denies preceding illnesses and has not been taking any new medications. Physical examination shows no lymphadenopathy or hepatosplenomegaly. Laboratory workup is significant for a hemoglobin of 6 g/dL, reticulocyte index of 0.5%, mean corpuscular volume of 97 fL, total leukocyte count of 2,300/μL, absolute neutrophil count of 1,100/μL, and platelet count of 12,000/μL. Bone marrow biopsy is obtained and no chromosomal abnormalities are detected. Peripheral blood smear and bone marrow biopsy are shown below.

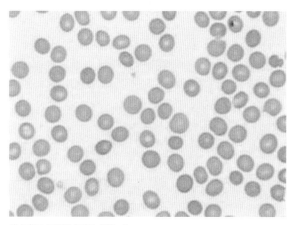

CASE FIGURE 30-1

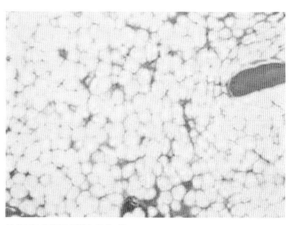

CASE FIGURE 30-2

QUESTION 1

★ What is the most likely diagnosis?

A. Aplastic anemia (AA)

B. Anemia of chronic disease (ACD)

C. Myelodysplastic syndrome (MDS)

D. Myeloproliferative neoplasm (MPN)

E. Autoimmune hemolytic anemia (AIHA)

Answer: A. Presentation with new onset pancytopenia, macrocytic anemia, low reticulocyte index, and bone marrow biopsy revealing hypocellularity is diagnostic of AA. Hypocellular MDS constitutes a minority of MDS cases, which typically exhibit hypercellularity. The presence of clonal chromosomal abnormalities, especially those typically observed in MDS, provides a strong argument for a diagnosis of MDS rather than AA (*Cancer*. 1988;62(5):958, *Br J Haematol*. 1995;91(3):612, *Exp Hematol*. 1987;15(11):1134).

QUESTION 2

☆ Testing for HIV and viral hepatitis and flow cytometry for paroxysmal nocturnal hemoglobinuria were negative. No culprit medications or chemicals were identified. There was no evidence of underlying autoimmune disorder or malignancy. What is the most appropriate management?

A. Reduced-intensity allogeneic hematopoietic stem cell transplantation

B. Rituximab

C. Cyclosporine

D. Antithymocyte globulin (ATG)

E. ATG and cyclosporine

Answer: E. Sibling-matched allogeneic stem cell transplantation is considered the first line of treatment in patients younger than 40 years, whereas immunosuppression with ATG and cyclosporine is considered for patients older than 40 years or those unable to undergo sibling-matched allogeneic hematopoietic stem cell transplantation for any reason. The use of matched unrelated donors or umbilical cord blood for transplantation in relapsed cases or those with no sibling donor are currently being investigated (*Ann Intern Med*. 1997;126(2):107, *Blood*. 1995;85(1):283).

QUESTION 3

☆ Which form of ATG is more effective in the management of AA?

A. Horse ATG (h-ATG)

B. Rabbit ATG (r-ATG)

C. Both have equal efficacy

D. There are no available data

Answer: A. Studies show that the use of h-ATG is associated with higher response rates and survival compared with r-ATG (*NEJM*. 2011;365(5):430, *Blood*. 2012;119(23):5391).

QUESTION 4

☆ Patient is treated appropriately with immunosuppression; however, 46 months later she presents to the emergency department complaining of severe abdominal pain. Evaluation revealed evidence of acute mesenteric venous thrombosis. What is the most appropriate next step in the management of this patient?

A. Test for JAK2 mutation

B. Test for factor V Leiden and prothrombin gene mutations

C. Flow cytometry for CD55 and CD59

D. Test for factor VIII level

E. Test for fibrinogen level

Answer: C. There is an increased risk of acquired clonal hematopoietic disorders in cases of AA; paroxysmal nocturnal hemoglobinuria (PNH), myelodysplastic syndrome, and acute myeloid leukemia. PNH clones are present in the majority of AA cases, either at diagnosis or later in the course of the disease. AA patients presenting with new venous thrombosis should be screened for PNH by using flow cytometry directed to the GPI-anchored proteins CD55 and CD59 (*Blood.* 1995;85(11):3058, *NEJM.* 1993;329(16):1152, *Blood.* 1995;85(5):1354, *Blood.* 1994;83(8):2323, *Haematologica.* 2010; 95(7):1075, *Ann Intern Med.* 1999;131(6):401, *Br J Haematol.* 1999;107(3):505).

CASE 31

A 57-year-old male is referred for further evaluation regarding generalized lymphadenopathy and leukocytosis. Patient reports generalized fatigue and night sweats for the preceding 2 months. Physical examination reveals bilateral cervical and axillary lymphadenopathy. No palpable hepatosplenomegaly is elicited. Laboratory workup shows leukocyte count of 38,000/μL, hemoglobin of 12.8 g/dL, and platelet count of 157,000/μL. Peripheral blood smear is shown below.

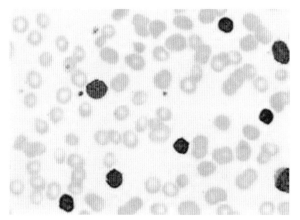

CASE FIGURE 31-1

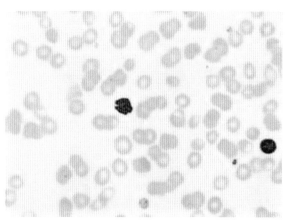

CASE FIGURE 31-2

Flow cytometry of peripheral blood is performed and reveals expression of CD10, CD19, and CD20 and lack of expression of CD5 and CD23. Bone marrow aspiration and biopsy are obtained. Bone marrow biopsy is shown below.

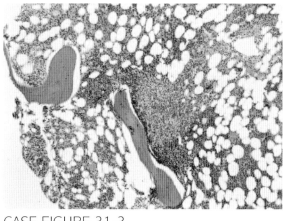

CASE FIGURE 31-3

QUESTION 1

✱ What is the most likely diagnosis?

A. Follicular lymphoma (FL)
B. Small lymphocytic lymphoma/chronic lymphocytic leukemia (SLL/CLL)
C. Hairy cell leukemia (HCL)
D. Mantle cell lymphoma (MCL)
E. Burkitt lymphoma/leukemia (BL)

Answer: A. Peripheral blood smear reveals increased number of mature-appearing lymphocytes with condensed chromatin and exhibiting nuclear clefts, "buttocks cells." Flow cytometry reveals lack of expression of CD5 and CD23 with positive expression of CD10, and bone marrow biopsy reveals a paratrabecular infiltrate characteristic of follicular lymphoma involvement. Bone marrow involvement is reported in 40% to 70% of patients with FL, and 33% also have peripheral blood involvement. Lack of CD5 and CD23 expression in addition to the pattern of bone marrow involvement make SLL/CLL less likely. MCL typically lacks expression of CD23 while being positive for CD5.

CASE 32

A 35-year-old male immigrant from Ghana presents for further evaluation of abnormal complete blood count obtained for health screening. Patient reports feeling well. Physical examination reveals minimal splenomegaly. Laboratory workup shows hemoglobin of 13.2 g/dL, red cell count (RBC) of 4.8 million/μL, mean corpuscular volume (MCV) of 74 fL, leukocyte count of 6,200/μL, and platelet count of 278,000/μL. Total bilirubin is minimally elevated at 1.6 mg/dL with a direct component of 0.3 mg/dL. Hemoglobin electrophoresis reveals no evidence of HbA and elevated HbF at 6%. Peripheral blood smear is shown below.

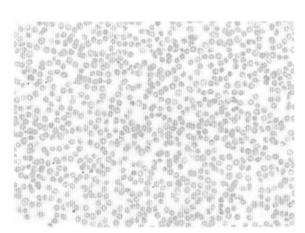

CASE FIGURE 32-1   CASE FIGURE 32-2

QUESTION 1

⭐ What is the most likely diagnosis?

A. Beta-thalassemia minor
B. Alpha-thalassemia trait
C. Hemoglobin C disease (homozygous, HbCC)
D. Hemoglobin E disease (homozygous, HbEE)
E. Hemoglobin C trait (heterozygous, HbAC)

Answer: C. Clinical presentation depicts an immigrant from West Africa presenting with minimal anemia, microcytosis, and evidence of hemolysis. Peripheral blood smear reveals evidence of codocytes (target-shaped RBCs) in addition to RBC with an uneven distribution of hemoglobin toward one portion of RBC (hemoglobin crystals). Hemoglobin electrophoresis reveals the presence of HbC (94%) and absence of HbA, with increased HbF levels. This is the classical presentation of HbC disease (HbCC). Hemoglobin beta chain mutation resulting in HbC is common in West Africa. Individuals with HbC trait (HbAC) are phenotypically normal, while those with HbC disease (HbCC) usually exhibit mild, compensated hemolytic anemia, splenomegaly, target RBCs, and HbC crystals that are formed secondary to decreased HbC solubility hemoglobin E disease and trait are common in populations of southeast Asia. (*Blood.* 1985;66(4):775, *Blood.* 2000;96(7):2358).

CASE 33

A 38-year-old male immigrant from Thailand is referred for further evaluation of progressive fatigue for the past 2 years. Physical examination discloses splenomegaly with no lymphadenopathy. Laboratory workup reveals hemoglobin of 8.2 g/dL, mean corpuscular volume (MCV) of 64 fL, leukocyte count of 4,900/μL, platelet count of 158,000/μL, and ferritin level of 462 ng/mL. Hemoglobin electrophoresis reveals HbE 58% and HbF 42%. Peripheral smear is shown below.

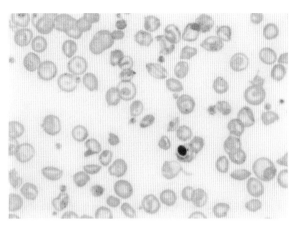

CASE FIGURE 33-1

QUESTION 1

☆ What is the most likely underlying disorder?

A. Hemoglobin E trait (heterozygous, HbAE)
B. HbE/beta^0-thalassemia
C. Hemoglobin E disease (homozygous, HbEE)
D. Sickle cell disease (HbSS)
E. HbS/beta-thalassemia

Answer: B. Peripheral slide reveals many target (codocytes)-shaped microcytic hypochromic red blood cells (RBC). There is no evidence of sickled RBCs. Elevated ferritin level rules out iron deficiency as a cause of the anemia. Hemoglobin E trait (heterozygous) cases usually present with normal hemoglobin, but exhibit mild microcytosis and hypochromia, and hemoglobin electrophoresis would reveal a smaller amount of HbE (30%), normal level of HbF, and HbA of 70%. Patients with hemoglobin E disease (homozygous) exhibit mild degree of anemia with microcytosis, hypochromia, and target cells. Hemoglobin electrophoresis reveals much higher HbE levels (90%). Cases of HbE/beta-thalassemia exhibit moderate to severe microcytosis with hypochromia and the presence of target cells. Hemoglobin electrophoresis shows elevated HbF levels (40%), with the remaining being HbE (60%). The etiology of the increased levels of HbF in HbE/beta^0-thalassemia appears to relate to survival advantage of erythroid progenitors committed to HbF synthesis in the highly stimulated bone marrow environment. Blood transfusions have been shown to decrease HbF levels relative to HbE by decreasing erythropoietin levels and bone marrow stimulation (*Blood.* 1999;94(9):3199, *Hematol Oncol Clin North Am.* 2010;24(6):1055, *Hematology Am Soc Hematol Educ Program.* 2007; Hemoglobin E Syndromes:79).

CASE 34

A 65-year-old male with a history of prostate cancer on hormonal therapy presents for evaluation of worsening fatigue and increasing bone pain. Physical examination reveals pallor and diffuse vertebral tenderness. Laboratory evaluation shows hemoglobin of 8.6 g/dL, leukocyte count of 22,600/μL, and platelet count of 58,000/μL. PSA is increased 597 ng/mL. Peripheral blood smear is shown below.

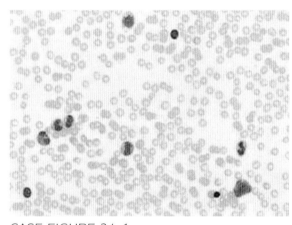

CASE FIGURE 34-1

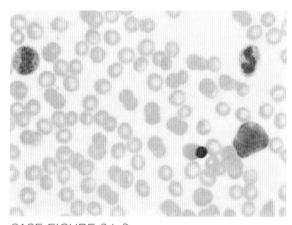

CASE FIGURE 34-2

QUESTION 1

☆ What is the most appropriate next step in management?

A. Discontinue hormonal therapy and initiate chemotherapy
B. Check testosterone levels
C. Check iron, folate, and vitamin B$_{12}$ levels
D. Flow cytometry of the peripheral blood
E. Bone marrow aspiration and biopsy

Answer: E. Peripheral slide reveals evidence of nucleated red blood cells (RBC) in addition to leukocytosis, with evidence of promyelocytes and metamyelocytes in peripheral blood and thrombocytopenia. This picture is concerning for an underlying bone marrow dysfunction and constitutes an indication for bone marrow evaluation. Leukoerythroblastosis is characterized by the presence in peripheral blood of RBCs exhibiting abnormal morphology: dacrocytes (tear drops), nucleated RBCs, and immature leukocytes, including occasional blasts and giant platelets. It is usually indicative of bone marrow replacement by an exogenous process.

QUESTION 2

Bone marrow biopsy is obtained and reveals extensive replacement of the normal hematopoietic elements by an infiltrating process as shown below.

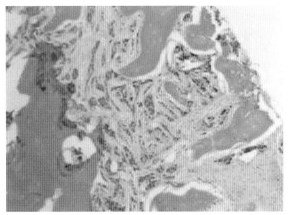

CASE FIGURE 34-3   CASE FIGURE 34-4

✯   What is the most likely diagnosis?

A. Myelophthisic anemia
B. Anemia of chronic disease
C. Aplastic anemia
D. Androgen deficiency
E. Autoimmune hemolytic anemia

Answer: A. Myelophthisic anemia results from bone marrow involvement by a pathological process resulting in replacement of the normal hematopoietic elements by metastatic tumor cells, granulomas, or marrow fibrosis. Leukoerythoblastic anemia is associated with the diagnosis of progressive and metastatic to bone hormone refractory prostate cancer in up to 30% of cases. Immunohistochemical stain for prostate specific antigen (PSA) confirmed a diagnosis of metastatic prostate cancer in this patient. (*Cancer.* 1979;44(3):1009, *Cancer.* 1993;71(11):3594, *Cancer.* 1983;51(2):308).

A 53-year-old female presents for evaluation of left-sided abdominal pain. Patient reports no weight loss, fever, or night sweats. Physical examination reveals massive splenomegaly extending into the pelvis with no lymphadenopathy. Laboratory workup shows leukocyte count of 5,900/μL, hemoglobin of 9.7 g/dL, and platelets of 97,000/μL. Peripheral smear is shown below.

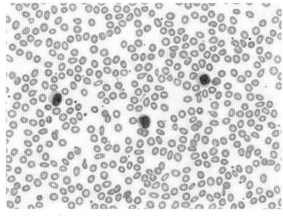

CASE FIGURE 35-1

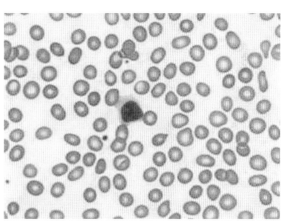

CASE FIGURE 35-2

Bone marrow biopsy shows involvement by multiple lymphoid aggregates as shown below.

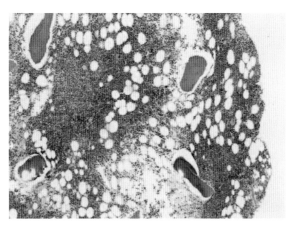

CASE FIGURE 35-3

PET/CT shows increased activity in the spleen. Flow cytometry of the peripheral blood reveals increased population of cells expressing CD20 but lacking the expression of CD5, CD10, and CD23.

QUESTION 1

⭐ What is the most likely diagnosis?

A. Follicular lymphoma (FL)
B. Mantle cell lymphoma (MCL)
C. Hairy cell leukemia (HCL)
D. Splenic marginal zone lymphoma (SMZL)
E. Small lymphocytic lymphoma/chronic lymphocytic leukemia (SLL/CLL)

Answer: D. The case presents a patient with bicytopenia, increased population of mature-appearing lymphocytes in peripheral blood with ample basophilic cytoplasm and condensed chromatin. Close examination of the surface of lymphocytes reveals the presence of small, irregularly distributed villous projections. Bone marrow biopsy exhibits nodular lymphoid aggregates, and flow cytometry reveals lack of expression of CD5, CD10, and CD23. This clinical presentation is most consistent with splenic marginal zone lymphoma, a subtype of marginal zone lymphoma. SMZL is uncommon, comprising about 2% to 5% of lymphomas. Patients present with splenomegaly, sometimes massive, with minimal or no peripheral lymphadenopathy. Hepatitis C has been described in association with SMZL. Lack of CD10 expression differentiates SMZL from FL, which is usually CD10 positive. Lack of expression of CD5 differentiates SMZL from MCL, and lack of CD5 and CD23 expression is useful in ruling out SLL/CLL. Nodular involvement of the bone marrow is useful in distinguishing SMZL from HCL, which usually presents with diffuse bone marrow involvement rather than a nodular pattern seen in SMZL (*Blood.* 2003;101(7):2464, *Br J Haematol.* 2003;122(3):404, *Blood.* 2002;100(5):1648, *Leukemia.* 2008;22(3):487, *Cancer.* 2004;101(9):2050).

CASE 36

A 69-year-old male is referred by his primary care physician for further evaluation of splenomegaly and abnormal peripheral blood counts. Patient reports a several-month history of progressive left abdominal discomfort and generalized fatigue. Physical examination confirms massive splenomegaly and reveals no lymphadenopathy. Laboratory noted a leukocyte count of 52,700/μL, hemoglobin of 11.3 g/dL, and platelet count of 120,000/μL. Peripheral blood count is shown below.

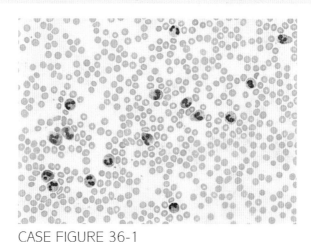

CASE FIGURE 36-1

Bone marrow aspiration and biopsy revealed hypercellular bone marrow, less than 5% blasts, and no evidence of dysplasia. Testing for *BCR-ABL* translocation was negative.

QUESTION 1

★ What is the most likely diagnosis?

A. Chronic lymphocytic leukemia (CLL)
B. Chronic neutrophilic leukemia (CNL)
C. Chronic myeloid leukemia (CML)
D. Atypical chronic myeloid leukemia (aCML)
E. Chronic myelomonocytic leukemia (CMML)

Answer: B. Peripheral blood smear reveals increased number of mature-appearing neutrophils with blue Dohle-like inclusions and lack of less-mature myeloid forms. There is no monocytosis. Bone marrow biopsy reveals lack of dysplasia and less than 5% myeloid blasts. Testing for *BCR-ABL* transcript was negative. This compilation of features is characteristic of CNL. Lack of increased monocyte count does not support the diagnosis of CMML, while negativity for *BCR-ABL* rules out CML. Atypical CML is defined as a *BCR-ABL* negative myeloproliferative/myelodysplastic syndrome, and characteristically exhibits dysplastic changes. Imatinib or other tyrosine kinase inhibitors do not have activity in cases of CNL. Lasting remissions have been reported with the use of interferon alfa (*Br J Haematol.* 2002;116(1):10, *Curr Hematol Rep.* 2004;3(3):210, *J Clin Pathol.* 2002;55(11):862, *J Clin Oncol.* 2001; 19(11):2915, *Ann Oncol.* 2000;11(4):441).

CASE 37

A 43-year-old male presents for further evaluation secondary to a 1-year history of chest pain, fatigue, generalized itching, and cough. Physical examination reveals hepatosplenomegaly. Laboratory studies show leukocyte count of 17,400/μL, absolute eosinophil count of 11,000/μL, hemoglobin 14.5 g/dL, and platelet count of 156,000/μL. Peripheral blood smear is shown below.

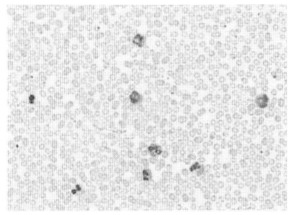

CASE FIGURE 37-1

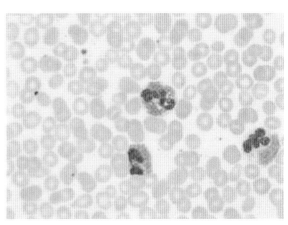

CASE FIGURE 37-2

Bone marrow aspiration and biopsy is obtained and reveales hypercellularity with increased eosinophil precursors.

QUESTION 1

☆ What is the most appropriate next step in management?

A. Test for *BCR*-ABL transcript
B. Test for 4q deletion
C. Test for 5q deletion
D. Choices A and B
E. Choices A, B, and C

Answer: D. The blood smear shows marked increase in eosinophils, some with vacuoles, sparse granulation, and nuclear hypersegmentation. It is noteworthy that there is no basophilia or myeloid left shift typical of chronic myeloid leukemia (CML). The two major differential diagnoses in this case are chronic myeloid leukemia (CML) presenting with associated eosinophilia PDGFRA associated myeloid neoplasm and chronic eosinophilic leukemia not otherwise specified (CEL-NOS). Testing for *BCR-ABL* transcript will help distinguish between the *BCR-ABL* positive CML and the other disorders. Interstitial deletion of chromosome 4q12 resulting in a chimeric fusion gene, *FIP1L1-PDGFRA*, is the most common chromosomal abnormality in cases presenting as CEL, and is detected in 14% of cases. This deletion affects the locus of *CHIC2* gene, and testing for *FIP1L1-PDGFRA* fusion is performed using FISH for *CHIC2* locus. By definition, CEL-NOS is negative for PDGFRA fusion gene (citation). (*Blood.* 2004;104(10):3038).

QUESTION 2

✭ Testing confirmed the presence of 4q12 deletion and absence of *BCR-ABL* translocation. What is the most appropriate management of this patient?

A. Imatinib
B. Cytarabine and daunorubicin (7 + 3 regimen)
C. Etoposide
D. Lenalidomide
E. Everolimus

Answer: A. Low-dose imatinib has demonstrated remarkable activity in cases of myeloid neoplasms harboring *PDGFRA* mutations or fusions, with more than 80% of cases achieving complete molecular remissions, and it is currently considered the first-line treatment. Cardiac involvement is the major cause of morbidity and mortality in these patients (*Br J Haematol.* 2008;143(5):707, *N Engl J Med.* 2003;348(13):1201, *Blood.* 2004;104(7):1931, *Blood.* 2007;109(11):4635, *Blood.* 2004;104(10):3038, *Blood.* 2003;101(12):4714, *Blood.* 2003;101(9):3391, *Haematologica.* 2007;92(9):1173, *Immunol Allergy Clin North Am.* 2007;27(3):457).

CASE 38

A 56-year-old female is referred by her primary care physician for further evaluation of life-long anemia. Patient reports that she required only a few red blood cell (RBC) transfusions during her life. Physical examination discloses splenomegaly. Laboratory workup reveals hemoglobin of 8.1 g/dL, mean corpuscular volume (MCV) of 106 fL, leukocyte count of 2,200/μL, and platelet count of 179,000/μL, with a ferritin level of 723 ng/mL. Old medical records are obtained, and reveal a hemoglobin of 9.5 g/dL, MCV of 103 fL, leukocyte count of 5,600/μL, and platelet count of 278,000/μL during her first year of life. Bone marrow aspirate is obtained and is shown below.

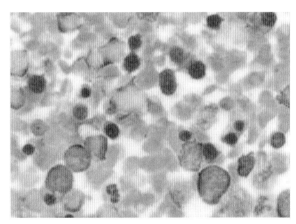 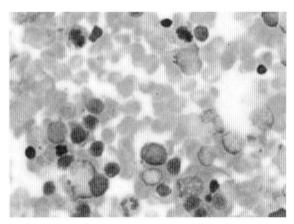

CASE FIGURE 38-1   CASE FIGURE 38-2

QUESTION 1

★ What is the most likely diagnosis?

A. Congenital dyserythropoietic anemia (CDA)
B. Myelodysplastic syndrome (MDS)
C. Aplastic anemia (AA)
D. Diamond Blackfan anemia (DBA)
E. Beta thalassemia major

Answer: A. CDA results in ineffective erythropoiesis and commonly manifests in the first decade of life with macrocytic anemia, the presence of multinucleated erythroblasts with erythroid hyperplasia, and nuclear chromatin bridges between erythroblasts in the bone marrow (noted in above images). Three different subclasses of CDA have been identified with distinct underlying genetic abnormalities and phenotypic features. Increased iron stores are present even without blood transfusions and are thought to be due to ineffective erythropoiesis and increased intestinal iron absorption. Mutations in codanin-1 may be involved in the pathogenesis of CDA type 1. Therapy depends on the subtype and includes splenectomy, interferon alfa, and judicious use of transfusions. The presence of macrocytic anemia since infancy and lack of dysplasia affecting other blood lineages strongly argues against MDS. Increased bone marrow cellularity and preserved leukocyte and platelet counts do not fit the diagnosis of AA. DBA is also characterized by macrocytic anemia that is usually evident in the first decade of life. However, bone marrow evaluation characteristically reveals the absence of erythroid precursors (*Curr Opin Hematol.* 2000;7(2):71, *Blood Rev.* 1998;12(3):178, *Am J Hematol.* 1996;51(1):55, *Blood.* 2008; 112(13):5241, *Br J Haematol.* 2005;131(4):431, *Curr Opin Hematol.* 2000;7(2):85).

CASE 39

A 76-year-old male presents for further evaluation of dyspnea and progressive erythematous rash on both lower extremities. Physical examination confirms the presence of erythematous plaques on both lower extremities in addition to disclosing hepatosplenomegaly and decreased breath sounds at both lung bases. Imaging shows bilateral moderate pleural effusions. Laboratory workup reveals hemoglobin of 8.6 g/dL, leukocyte count of 173,000/μL, and platelet count of 98,000/μL. Flow cytometry reveals expression of CD2, CD3, CD4, CD5, CD7, and CD52, with lack of CD8 expression. Peripheral slide is shown below.

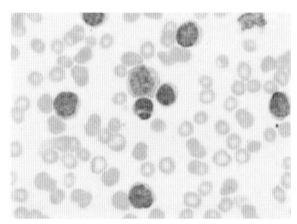

CASE FIGURE 39-1

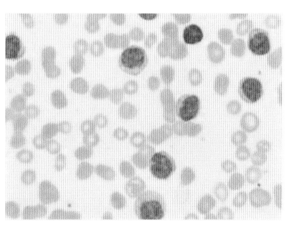

CASE FIGURE 39-2

QUESTION 1

⭐ What is the most likely diagnosis?

A. Chronic lymphocytic leukemia (CLL)
B. T-cell prolymphocytic leukemia (T-PLL)
C. B-cell prolymphocytic leukemia (B-PLL)
D. T-cell large granular lymphocyte leukemia (T-LGL)
E. Mantle cell lymphoma (MCL)

Answer: B. Peripheral blood examination reveals the presence of increased number of lymphoid cells that are characteristically larger than their normal counterparts and exhibit condensed chromatin and the presence of single nucleoli in addition to increased amount of basophilic cytoplasm lacking granulation. Flow cytometry shows expression of T-cell markers, and thus rules out MCL, B-PLL, and CLL. The lack of cytoplasmic granulation argues against the diagnosis of T-LGL. T-PLL is a rare postthymic T-cell neoplasm. Hepatoplenomegaly is a common presenting manifestation. T-PLL is known to be associated with serous effusions and skin infiltration in up to 20% of cases. Skin lesions include nodules, rash, and erythroderma. CLL is a B-cell malignancy; however, a small case series describing 25 cases of what appeared to be T-cell CLL was reported. The abnormal lymphocytes did not exhibit the typical phenotype of prolymphocytes and thus did not meet diagnostic criteria for T-PLL. Whether these cases do represent rare cases of T-CLL or nonclassical T-PLL is not entirely clear. The prognosis of T-PLL is poor, with no clearly defined treatment regimens. Alemtuzumab and pentostatin have been used with response rates in excess of 50%; however, the duration of response is characteristically short (*Blood.* 1995;86(3):1163, *Mayo Clin Proc.* 2005;80(12):1660, *J Clin Oncol.* 2002;20(1):205, *Blood.* 2001;98(6):1721, *J Clin Oncol.* 2009;27(32):5425, *J Clin Oncol.* 1994;12(12): 2588, *Blood.* 2012;120(3):538).

CASE 40

A 57-year-old female is admitted to the hospital secondary to weakness, fatigue, and anorexia. Physical examination discloses massive splenomegaly with no evidence of lymphadenopathy or hepatomegaly. Laboratory workup reveals leukocyte count of 274,000/μL, hemoglobin of 8.2 g/dL, and platelet count of 85,000/μL. Flow cytometry shows increased population of cells expressing CD19, CD20, and surface IgM. Expression of CD5 and CD23 is absent. Peripheral blood smear is shown below.

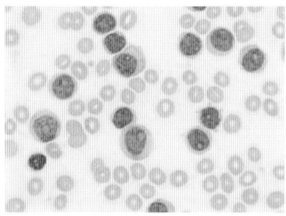 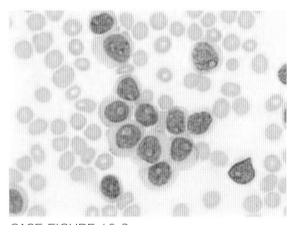

CASE FIGURE 40-1　　　　　　　　CASE FIGURE 40-2

QUESTION 1

☆ What is the most likely diagnosis?

A. Chronic lymphocytic leukemia (CLL)
B. T-cell prolymphocytic leukemia (T-PLL)
C. B-cell prolymphocytic leukemia (B-PLL)
D. T-cell large granular lymphocyte leukemia (T-LGL)
E. Mantle cell lymphoma (MCL)

Answer: C. Peripheral blood smear reveals that the majority of peripheral blood lymphocytes are larger in size than their normal counterparts, with ample amount of cytoplasm lacking granulation and prominent nucleoli. This finding and the immunophenotype are characteristic of B-PLL. B-PLL is a *de novo* leukemia in which prolymphocytes comprise 55% or more of the blood lymphocytes. Massive splenomegaly and systemic B symptoms are common presenting manifestations in patients with

B-PLL. Flow cytometry reveals lack of T-cell markers and lack of CD5 and CD23 expression. Lack of CD5 and CD23 expression is not consistent with classical CLL, while the lack of CD5 expression argues against the diagnosis of MCL. Absence of T-cell markers and cytoplasmic granulation does not support the diagnosis of T-LGL or T-PLL. Cases of B-PLL are characterized by strong expression of surface IgM. There is no standard regimen for the treatment of B-PLL; however, fludarabine, rituximab, and alemtuzumab in addition to classical combination chemotherapy regimens have been used with variable success (*Hematol Oncol Clin North Am.* 1990;4(2):457, *Hematol J.* 2004;5 Suppl 1:S50, *Leuk Lymphoma.* 2002;43(5):1007, *Am J Hematol.* 2007;82(5):417, *Ann Hematol.* 2004;83(5)319, *Blood.* 2012;120(3):538, *Leuk Lymphoma.* 1999;33(1–2):169).

QUESTION 2

✭ What is the most common chromosomal abnormality in cases of B-PLL?

A. del(17p)
B. t(11;14)
C. del(11q)
D. t(14;18)
E. del(5q)

Answer: A. Deletions of chromosome 17p affecting *p53* locus is seen in more than 50% of B-PLL cases. Presence of t(11;14) indicates the presence of MCL in leukemic phase, while t(14;18) is characteristic of but not diagnostic of follicular lymphoma (*Blood.* 1997;89(6)2015, *Br J Haematol.* 2004;125(3):330).

A 67-year-old female is referred for evaluation of chronic anemia and thrombocytopenia. Physical examination reveals no lymphadenopathy or hepatosplenomegaly. Laboratory evaluation shows hemoglobin of 9.7 g/dL, mean corpuscular volume of 104 fL, leukocyte count of 5,800/μL, and platelet count of 64,000/μL. Peripheral blood smear is shown below.

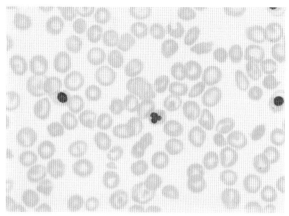

CASE FIGURE 41-1

Bone marrow aspiration revealed 2% blasts, and a sample of bone marrow aspirate is shown below.

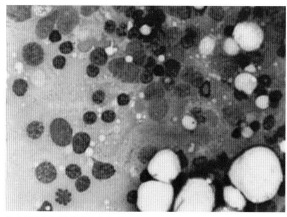

CASE FIGURE 41-2

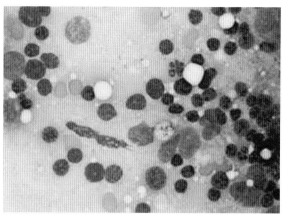

CASE FIGURE 41-3

QUESTION 1

✩ What is the most likely diagnosis?

A. Refractory cytopenia with unilineage dysplasia (RCUD)
B. Refractory anemia with excess blasts (RAEB)
C. 5q- syndrome
D. Acute myeloid leukemia (AML)
E. Myelofibrosis

Answer: A. Peripheral blood smear reveals anisopoikilocytosis and the presence of nucleated red blood cell (RBC) precursors, one with nuclear budding, with absent blasts. Bone marrow biopsy reveals hypercellularity, and the aspirate demonstrates abnormal RBC progenitors exhibiting multinucleation, nuclear budding, and abnormal nuclear forms. Bone marrow blast count is less than 5%, with absence of significant dysplastic changes in other hematopoietic lineages. This is the classic presentation of refractory anemia with unilineage dysplasia (RCUD). Refractory anemia constitutes 21% of newly diagnosed cases of MDS and is characterized by low risk of progression to AML. Cases of 5q- syndrome classically present with female predominance, preserved leukocyte and platelet counts, and thrombocytosis with increased number of abnormal hypolobated micromegarakyocytes (*Blood.* 2004;103(9):3265, *Blood.* 2002;100(7):2292, *Blood.* 2009;113(25):6296, *J Clin Oncol.* 2007;25(23):3503).

A 58-year-old male presents for further evaluation of anemia. Physical examination reveals no lymphadenopathy or hepatosplenomegaly. Laboratory workup shows hemoglobin 7.7 g/dL, mean corpuscular volume 104 fL, leukocyte count 7,800/μL, and platelet count 760,000/μL. Ferritin level is elevated. Peripheral blood smear is shown below.

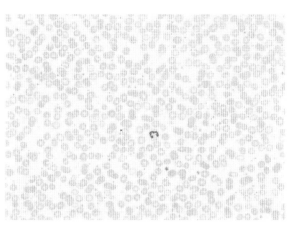

CASE FIGURE 42-1

Bone marrow aspirate and Prussian blue iron stain of bone marrow aspirate are shown below.

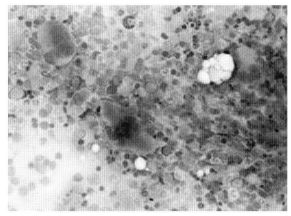

CASE FIGURE 42-2

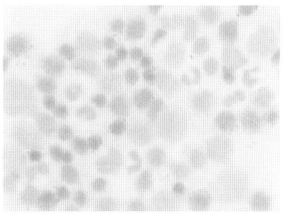

CASE FIGURE 42-3

QUESTION 1

✶ What test(s) are considered appropriate for the evaluation of this case?

A. Testing for JAK2 mutation
B. Testing for *BCR-ABL* translocation
C. Cytogenetics
D. All of the above
E. None of the above

Answer: D. Peripheral smear reveals evidence of anisopoikilocytosis, platelets exhibiting different sizes and abnormal granulation, and a hypogranular neutrophil. Macrocytic anemia and increased number of ring sideroblasts in the bone marrow, evident with Prussian blue stain, are characteristic of refractory anemia with ring sideroblasts (RARS). Thrombocytosis is a rare feature of newly diagnosed myelodysplastic syndrome (MDS). It has been associated with 5q- syndrome, 3q syndrome, and cases otherwise meeting criteria for RARS. Ruling out an underlying myeloproliferative disorder (MPD) or chronic myeloid leukemia is also appropriate in the workup of this case (*Luek Lymphoma.* 2007;48(12):2375, *Haematologica.* 1999;84(8):690, *Leuk Lymphoma.* 2003;44(3):557).

QUESTION 2

✶ Evaluation revealed absence of BCR-ABL translocation. Cytogenetics revealed no abnormalities. JAK2 mutation was present. What is the most likely diagnosis?

A. Refractory anemia with ring sideroblasts (RARS)
B. Refractory anemia with ring sideroblasts and thrombocytosis (RARS-T)
C. Essential thrombocytosis
D. 5q- syndrome
E. 3q syndrome

Answer: B. Refractory anemia with ring sideroblasts and thrombocytosis (RARS-T) is considered to represent an overlap syndrome between myelodysplastic (RARS) and myeloproliferative syndromes. This notion is supported by the presence of JAK2 mutation in 67% of cases meeting criteria for RARS-T (*Leuk Lymphoma.* 2003; 44(3):557, *Leuk Lymphoma.* 1999;34(5–6):615, *Br J Haematol.* 2009;144(6):809, *Blood.* 2006;108(7):2173, *Blood.* 2007;109(3):1334).

CASE 43

A 68-year-old male presents for further evaluation of fatigue and dyspnea on exertion. Physical examination reveals no hepatosplenomegaly or lymphadenopathy. Laboratory workup reveals leukocyte count of 67,000/μL, hemoglobin of 6.4 g/dL, and platelet count of 262,000/μL. Flow cytometry of peripheral blood is performed and reveals expression of CD5, CD19, CD20, and CD23. Peripheral slide is shown below.

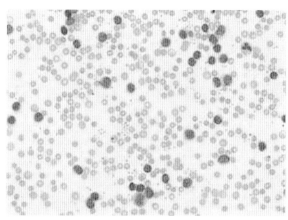

CASE FIGURE 43-1

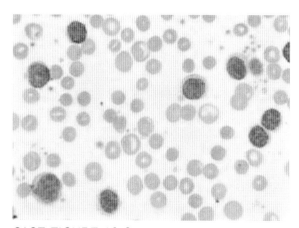

CASE FIGURE 43-2

QUESTION 1

✶ What is the most likely underlying diagnosis?

A. Mantle cell lymphoma (MCL)
B. Chronic lymphocytic leukemia (CLL)
C. Follicular lymphoma (FL)
D. Chronic myeloid leukemia (CML)
E. T-cell prolymphocytic leukemia (T-PLL)

Answer: B. Peripheral blood smear reveals increased number of mature-appearing lymphocytes with clumped chromatin and small amount of cytoplasm. Flow cytometry reveals the typical signature of CLL with expression of CD5, CD20, and CD23. Presence of CD5 rules out the diagnosis of FL, while expression of CD23 argues against MCL. Minority of the lymphocytes are of a larger size; however, they do not exhibit prominent nucleoli characteristic of prolymphocytes. Absence of the usual T-cell markers rules out the diagnosis of T-PLL.

QUESTION 2

✶   What is the most likely etiology of anemia in this case?

A. Autoimmune hemolytic anemia (AIHA)
B. Bone marrow infiltration by CLL
C. Pure red blood cell aplasia (PRCA)
D. Hypersplenism
E. Anemia of chronic disease

Answer: A. Peripheral blood smear reveals spherocytes and reticulocytosis, suggesting increased bone marrow production of red blood cells (RBC) to compensate for the anemia. This argues against bone marrow infiltration by CLL, PRCA, and anemia of chronic disease, as all of these entities are characterized by suppressed bone marrow function. Hypersplenism is less likely in the absence of splenomegaly. AIHA appears to be a relatively uncommon feature of the natural history of CLL, occurring in less than 10% of cases throughout their disease course. AIHA does not appear to impact the prognosis or the outcome of treatment. The distinction between anemia caused by bone marrow infiltration by CLL and AIHA is essential for treatment. The management of AIHA associated with CLL follows the usual algorithm for the management of idiopathic AIHA. In cases of refractory AIHA, treatment of underlying CLL is indicated (*Blood.* 2000;95(9):2786, *Br J Haematol.* 1987;67(2):235, *Br J Haematol.* 2011;154(1):14, *Blood.* 2010;115(2):187).

CASE 44

A 20-year-old college student presents for evaluation of anemia. Patient reports a history of sore throat 2 weeks previously. Physical examination reveals bilateral cervical lymphadenopathy and mild splenomegaly. Laboratory studies note a leukocyte count of 11,200/μL, hemoglobin 8.7 g/dL, mean corpuscular volume (MCV) 108 fL, and platelet count of 250,000/μL. Peripheral blood smear is shown below. Monospot testing is positive.

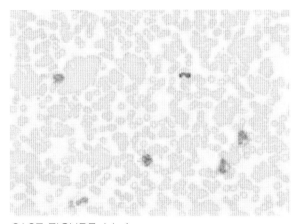

CASE FIGURE 44-1

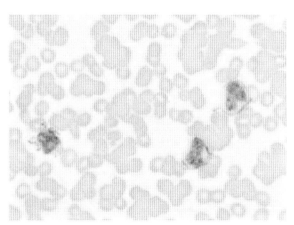

CASE FIGURE 44-2

QUESTION 1

★ What is the most likely diagnosis?

A. Warm autoimmune hemolytic anemia (AIHA)
B. Cold agglutinin induced hemolysis
C. Vitamin B$_{12}$ deficiency
D. Paroxysmal nocturnal hemoglobinuria (PNH)
E. Acute lymphoblastic leukemia (ALL)

Answer: B. Peripheral blood smear demonstrates the presence of reactive lymphocytes and red blood cell (RBC) agglutination, which results in spurious elevation of MCV. Cold agglutinin-induced hemolysis is characterized by the presence of IgM antibodies directed against the RBC "I" or "i" antigen. The underlying etiology can range from benign conditions like infections (infectious mononucleosis or mycoplasma pneumoniae) to aggressive lymphomas. The cause of anemia is extravascular hemolysis. Treatment options range from cold avoidance to rituximab, cytotoxic chemotherapy, or plasma exchange for rapid removal of IgM from the circulation. Contrary to their benefit in the management of warm AIHA, corticosteroids have no proven benefit in the treatment of cold agglutinin disease (*Blood.* 1977;50(2):195, *Br J Haematol.* 2011;153(3):309, *Br J Haematol.* 2007;138(4):422).

CASE 45

A 32-year-old female with no known medical problems is referred for further evaluation of new onset anemia and thrombocytopenia. Physical examination reveals no lymphadenopathy or hepatosplenomegaly. Laboratory workup shows hemoglobin 7.6 g/dL, leukocyte count 4,500/μL, and platelet count 7,000/μL. Direct antiglobin test is positive for IgG. LDH was elevated at 370 U/L. Testing for HIV and viral hepatitis is negative. Peripheral blood smear is shown below.

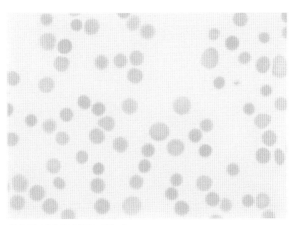

CASE FIGURE 45-1

QUESTION 1

⭐ What is the most likely diagnosis?

A. Evans syndrome (ES)
B. Felty syndrome (FS)
C. Autoimmune hemolytic anemia (AIHA)
D. Immune thrombocytopenic purpura (ITP)
E. Myelophthisic anemia

Answer: A. Peripheral slide reveals the presence of spherocytes and reticulocytosis, which in the context of direct antiglobin test positivity and elevated LDH is consistent with the diagnosis of AIHA. There is no clear underlying etiology of thrombocytopenia, and given the presence of AIHA, it is very likely caused by immune destruction, ITP. The combination of AIHA and ITP is referred to as ES. FS is characterized by the presence of rheumatoid arthritis, neutropenia, and splenomegaly. Absence of leukoerythroblastosis in peripheral blood argues against the presence of myelophthisic anemia. ES can present as a primary disorder or occur in context of another autoimmune condition. Management follows the algorithm for AIHA and ITP with the use of corticosteroids, splenectomy, rituximab, or other immunosuppressive agents. The course of ES tends to be more aggressive than that of either AIHA or ITP, and is characterized by a chronic course with frequent relapses (*Blood.* 2009;114(15):3167, *Br J Haematol.* 2006;132(2):125).

A 59-year-old female with prior medical history significant for systemic lupus erythe-matosus (SLE) treated with methotrexate is seen for symptoms of nausea, vomiting, and diarrhea for the preceding week not responding to antibiotic therapy. Laboratory workup reveals leukocyte count of 4,600/μL, hemoglobin 7.9 g/dL, and platelet count 3,000/μL. There is evidence of acute renal insufficiency and marked liver enzyme eleva-tion, LDH 2,078 U/L, triglycerides 700 mg/dL, and ferritin 17,285 ng/mL. Coagulation parameters reveal PT of 14 seconds, PTT of 59 seconds, and hypofibrinogenemia. Bone marrow aspirate is obtained and is shown below.

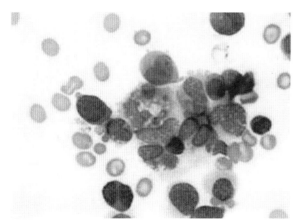 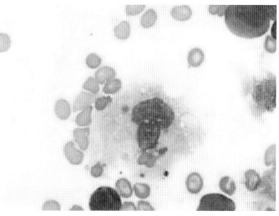

CASE FIGURE 46-1   CASE FIGURE 46-2

QUESTION 1

✫ What is the most likely explanation of her presentation?

A. Macrophage activation syndrome (MAS)
B. Methotrexate induced bone marrow suppression
C. Evans syndrome (ES)
D. SLE-associated aplastic anemia
E. Felty syndrome (FS)

Answer: A. Bone marrow aspirate reveals hemophagocytosis: macrophages engulfing leukocytes and red blood cells. MAS is a severe and life-threatening deregulation of the immune system that usually occurs on the background of preexisting autoimmune condition (SLE, RA) and is most commonly precipitated by infections or therapeutic manipulations. It is characterized by uncontrolled activation of macrophages and T-cells resulting in uncontrolled immune system stimulation. MAS is considered to represent a secondary or acquired form of hemophagocytic lymphohistiocytosis (HLH), and both conditions share several genetic alterations that result in decreased natural killer (NK) and cytotoxic T-cell activity. Classical laboratory features include pancytopenia, hypertriglyceridemia, hypofibrinogenemia, and marked hyperferritinemia (*Curr Opin Rheumatol.* 2010;22(5):561, *Curr Opin Rheumatol.* 2003;15(5):587, *Blood.* 2005;105(4):1648).

CASE 47

A 34-year-old female with anorexia nervosa (AN) is referred by her primary care physician for further evaluation of anemia and thrombocytopenia. Physical examination reveals an underweight and malnourished young female in no acute distress. Laboratory workup shows leukocyte count 9,000/μL, hemoglobin 7.9 g/dL, mean corpuscular volume (MCV) 101 fL, and platelet count 60,000/μL. Peripheral blood smear confirms the presence of thrombocytopenia, but shows no other gross abnormalities. Bone marrow biopsy is obtained and is shown below.

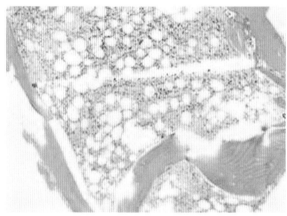

CASE FIGURE 47-1

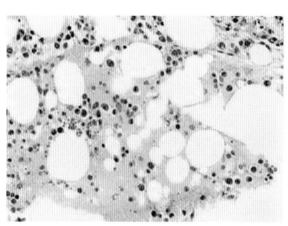

CASE FIGURE 47-2

QUESTION 1

⭐ What is the most likely explanation for her presentation?

A. Aplastic anemia (AA)
B. Folate deficiency
C. Vitamin B$_{12}$ deficiency
D. Gelatinous degeneration
E. Myelofibrosis (MF)

Answer: D. Bone marrow biopsy reveals the presence of an amorphous gelatinous eosinophilic infiltrate that replaces the normal hematopoietic elements. Hematologic abnormalities are common in patients with AN, and gelatinous degeneration of bone marrow has been reported in 50% of cases. AA would not be expected to exhibit the abnormal bone marrow infiltrate seen in this case. Although vitamin B_{12} and folate deficiencies are possible, they would not account for the bone marrow picture. MF presents with evidence of leukoerythroblastosis in the peripheral blood, and the bone marrow infiltrate seen in this case is not characteristic of bone marrow fibrosis seen with MF (*Int J Eat Disord.* 2009;42(4):293, *Am J Clin Pathol.* 2002;118(4):582, *Arch Intern Med.* 2005;165(5):561).

CASE 48

A 24-year-old Amish female is referred for evaluation of anemia. Patient states she had a splenectomy as a child for anemia, and other siblings also underwent splenectomy. Physical examination reveals no lymphadenopathy. Laboratory evaluation is significant for hemoglobin 9.2 g/dL, mean corpuscular volume (MCV) 121 fL, leukocyte count 7,400/μL, and platelet count 565,000/μL. Direct antiglobin test is negative. LDH is mildly elevated with decreased haptoglobin level. Peripheral slide is shown below.

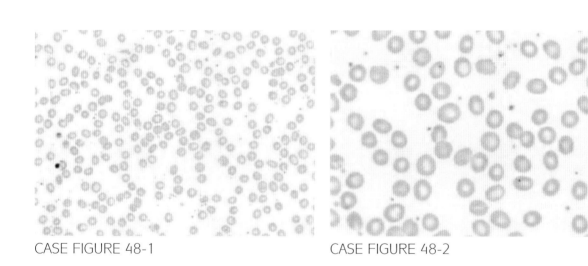

CASE FIGURE 48-1   CASE FIGURE 48-2

QUESTION 1

★ What is the most likely diagnosis?

A. Autoimmune hemolytic anemia (AIHA)
B. Hereditary spherocytosis (HS)
C. Pyruvate kinase deficiency (PK deficiency)
D. Iron-deficiency anemia
E. Vitamin B$_{12}$ deficiency

Answer: C. Peripheral blood smear reveals increased reticulocytes, echinocytes (burr cells), nucleated RBC, and Howell–Jolly bodies. There is no evidence of spherocytes and RBC exhibit normochromia with macrocytosis. The clinical picture in context with the patient's social and cultural background

111

is most consistent with PK deficiency-associated hemolytic anemia. PK deficiency is common in the Amish population and has been traced to a single founder mutation. Absence of spherocytes argues against the diagnosis of HS. This feature, in addition to a negative direct antiglobin test, rules out AIHA. Normochromia with macrocytosis are not consistent with the diagnosis of iron-deficiency anemia. While vitamin B_{12} deficiency can result in anemia, patient with such a degree of deficiency would be expected to exhibit variable levels of leukopenia and thrombocytopenia. Confirming low levels of PK activity is essential for the correct diagnosis (*J Clin Pathol*. 1999;52(4):241, *Br J Haematol*. 2005;130(1):11, *Blood*. 1994; 83: 2311).

A 31-year-old female presents with complaints of generalized weakness and progressively worsening pain in her left arm. Patient reports sustaining a bite on her left arm 5 days previously. On review of systems, patient admits having dark colored urine for the last 3 days. Physical examination reveals pallor and erythematous patch on the lateral aspect of her left arm with two blood-filled vesicles. Laboratory workup reveals leukocyte count of 42,500/μL, hemoglobin 4 g/dL, and platelet count 141,000/μL. Reticulocyte count is elevated. Direct antiglobin test is positive for both IgG and complement. LDH is 2,080 U/L, total bilirubin 9.1 mg/dL, and indirect bilirubin 8.2 mg/dL. Coagulation parameters are normal. Peripheral blood smear and left arm bite is shown below.

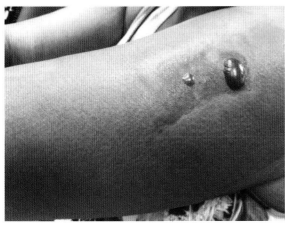

CASE FIGURE 49-1

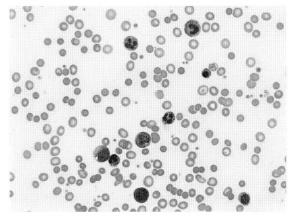

CASE FIGURE 49-2

QUESTION 1

★ What is the most likely explanation of her presentation?

A. Idiopathic immune hemolytic anemia
B. Loxoscelism
C. Paroxysmal nocturnal hemoglobinuria
D. Spherocytosis
E. G6PD deficiency-associated hemolysis

Answer: **B.** Peripheral slide demonstrates spherocytosis and increased reticulocytes. Leukocytes exhibit toxic granulation and vacuolation. Loxoscelism is a syndrome produced by the bite of *Loxosceles reclusa*, the brown recluse spider. Hematologic manifestations include disseminated intravascular coagulation and both intravascular and extravascular hemolysis with positive direct antiglobin test. Treatment is mainly supportive with red blood cell transfusions and corticosteroids (*Transfusion.* 2004;44(11):1543, *J Pediatr.* 2010;156(1):155, *Lancet.* 2011;378(9808):2039, *Cutis.* 2004;74(6):341, *Am J Med Sci.* 1992;304(4):261, *Am J Clin Pathol.* 1995;104(4):463).

CASE 50

A 22-year-old female graduate student from Africa presents with complaints of chills and fever for the past 2 days. Physical examination reveals fever of 104 °F and spleno-megaly. Laboratory workup shows leukocyte count of 7,800/μL, hemoglobin 8.7 g/dL, and platelet count 110,000/μL. Direct antiglobin test is negative. Peripheral blood smear is shown below.

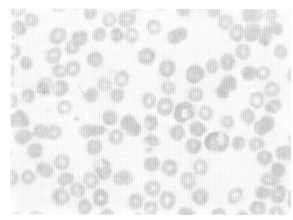

CASE FIGURE 50-1

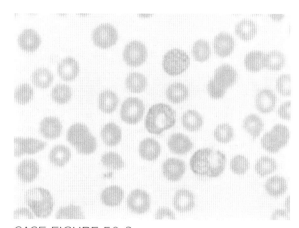

CASE FIGURE 50-2

QUESTION 1

★ What is the most likely diagnosis?

A. G6PD deficiency induced anemia
B. Hemoglobin C disease (homozygous, HbCC)
C. Hemoglobin H disease (HbH disease)
D. Malarial anemia
E. Hereditary spherocytosis (HS)

Answer: D. Peripheral smear reveals schizonts and gametocytes, which occupy almost the entire erythrocyte. This picture is most likely consistent with *Plasmodium vivax* infection. The presence of parasite-filled RBCs argues strongly against other diagnoses. There is no evidence of spherocytes to support the diagnosis of HS. Cases with HbH disease would reveal severe microcytosis and the pres-ence of target RBCs. Patients with HbC disease would also be expected to exhibit target RBCs and the characteristic RBC crystals. The clinical presentation, especially with high fever, is not consistent with the diagnosis of G6PD deficiency.

115

A 56-year-old male presents for further evaluation of fatigue. Physical examination reveals no lymphadenopathy or hepatosplenomegaly. Laboratory workup shows leukocyte count 17,300/μL, hemoglobin 8.2 g/dL, and platelet count 138,000/μL, in addition to new-onset renal failure and elevated LDH of 540 U/L. Peripheral slide reveals predominance of lymphoid appearing cells accounting for 40% of the leukocyte count as shown below.

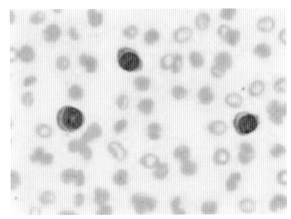

CASE FIGURE 51-1

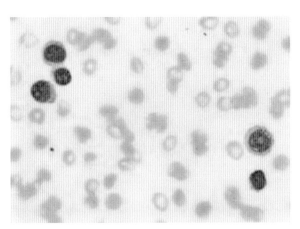

CASE FIGURE 51-2

Flow cytometry of peripheral blood is obtained and reveals increased population of cells expressing CD38 and CD138, with lack of CD56. Bone marrow aspiration is obtained and is shown below.

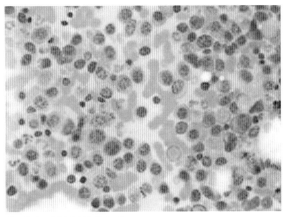

CASE FIGURE 51-3

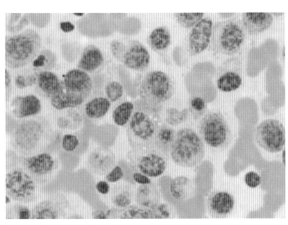

CASE FIGURE 51-4

QUESTION 1

✷ What is the most likely diagnosis?

A. Chronic lymphocytic leukemia (CLL)
B. Multiple myeloma (MM)
C. Plasma cell leukemia (PCL)
D. Acute lymphoblastic leukemia (ALL)
E. Acute myeloid leukemia (AML)

Answer: C. Peripheral blood and bone marrow reveals the presence of cells characterized by their oval shape, basophilic cytoplasm, eccentric nucleus, and perinuclear cytoplasmic clearing. Some of the cells exhibit higher nuclear-to-cytoplasmic ratios, dispersed chromatin, and prominent nucleoli consistent with immature plasma cell precursors. Flow cytometry reveals the typical plasma cell markers, CD38 and CD138, with absence of lymphoid or myeloid markers that would be typical of CLL, ALL, or AML. Lack of CD56 expression is characteristic to PCL as compared to MM. PCL can present as a primary condition with no antecedent MM, or more commonly evolve from a preceding MM. The diagnosis of PCL is established when the total number of circulating monoclonal plasma cells exceeds 2,000/μL or 20% of the total leukocyte count. Thus, in this case, the diagnosis of PCL is more appropriate than that of MM. The prognosis of PCL is poor, likely secondary to increased prevalence of high-risk cytogenetics. There is no standard treatment regimen, and combinations chemotherapy used for high-risk MM are commonly utilized in addition to hematopoietic stem cell transplantation. Enrolment into clinical trials is strongly recommended for appropriate patients (*Ann Oncol* 2011;22(7):1628, *Cancer* 2009;115(24):5734, *Leukemia* 2008;22(5):1044).

A 41-year-old female presents for further evaluation of several months of easy bruising. Physical examination reveals generalized patechiae with no hepatosplenomegaly or lymphadenopathy. Laboratory workup reveals leukocyte count 7,000/μL, hemoglobin 13.4 g/dL, and platelet 8,000/μL. Peripheral blood smear is shown below.

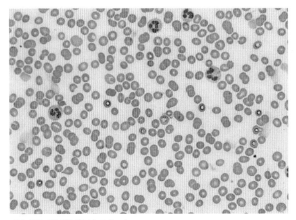

CASE FIGURE 52-1

Patient is diagnosed with immune thrombocytopenic purpura (ITP) and started on prednisone. On a follow-up visit 2 and 4 weeks later, there is no improvement in platelet count. Bone marrow aspiration and biopsy is obtained and is shown below.

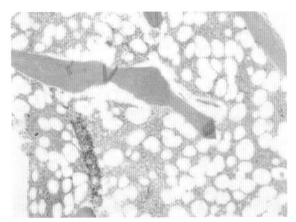

CASE FIGURE 52-2

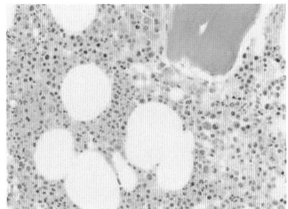

CASE FIGURE 52-3

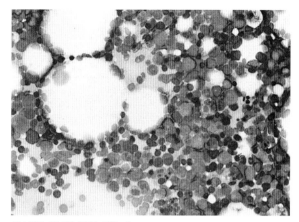

CASE FIGURE 52-4

QUESTION 1

☆ What is the most likely diagnosis?

A. Refractory ITP
B. Acute megakaryoblastic leukemia (AMKL)
C. Amegakaryocytic thrombocytopenia (AMT)
D. Aplastic anemia (AA)
E. Myelofibrosis (MF)

Answer: C. Peripheral blood smear reveals severe thrombocytopenia, with no abnormalities in leukocytes and RBCs. Failue of ITP to respond to corticosteroid therapy is usually considered an indication to perform bone marrow evaluation to rule out other pathology. Bone marrow aspirate and biopsy reveal absence of megakaryocytes, a finding not consistent with the diagnosis of ITP. This presentation is most consistent with acquired AMT, a condition characterized by the presence of pathologic autoantibodies directed at thrombopoietin receptor. Acquired AMT has been associated with other autoimmune conditions and large granular lymphocyte leukemia (LGL). Bone marrow biopsy and otherwise normal peripheral blood counts do not support the diagnosis of AA. There is no peripheral blood features or any evidence of marrow fibrosis that would be expected in cases of MF or AMKL. Treatment includes immunosuppression with cyclosporine, antithymocyte globulin, rituximab, or the use of thrombopoietin (TPO) agonist. Allogeneic hematopoietic stem cell transplantation has been used in few cases with durable responses (*Arthritis Rheum.* 2002;46(8):2148, Arthritis Rheum 2003;48(6):1647, *Am J Hematol.* 1999;62(2):115, *Am J Hematol.* 2007;82(7):650, *Clin Adv Hematol Oncol.* 2010;8(11):806, *Bone Marrow Transplant.* 1999;24(12):1337).

CASE 53

A 66-year-old male is referred for further evaluation of leukocytosis. Patient reports fatigue and left upper quadrant discomfort for several months. Physical examination reveals no lymphadenopathy but uncovers massive splenomegaly. Laboratory evaluation shows leukocyte count 62,800/μL, hemoglobin 6.2 g/dL, and platelet count 142,000/μL. Flow cytometry shows increased population of cells expressing CD11c, CD20, and CD103, and lacking expression of CD25, CD123, TRAP, and Annexin A1. Peripheral smear is shown below.

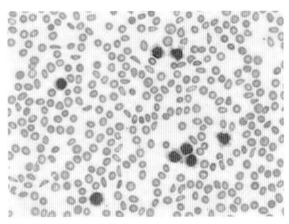 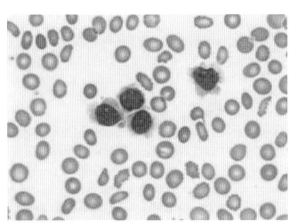

CASE FIGURE 53-1   CASE FIGURE 53-2

QUESTION 1

☆ What is the most likely diagnosis?

A. Chronic lymphocytic leukemia (CLL)
B. Mantle cell lymphoma (MCL)
C. Hairy cell leukemia variant (vHCL)
D. Follicular lymphoma
E. Splenic marginal zone lymphoma

Answer: C. Peripheral slide demonstrates the presence of large lymphocytes with irregular cytoplasmic projections and prominent nucleoli. Flow cytometry reveals expression of several markers characteristic of HCL, including CD11c, CD20, and CD103. Negativity for CD25, CD123, TRAP, and Annexin A1 in addition to easily obtainable bone marrow aspirate differentiates the classical and variant forms of HCL. The variant form of HCL tends to present with leukocytosis, rather than with pancytopenia, as seen in the classical form. The nucleoli are classically absent in the classic form as compared to prominent in the variant form of HCL. Overexpression of Annexin A1 gene distinguishes the two forms of HCL as well as differentiating classical HCL from other forms of lymphomas. Treatment regimens used for the classical form of HCL appear to be less effective when applied to the variant form. Data suggest that monoclonal antibodies have superior outcomes as compared to purine analogue regimens used for classical HCL (*Blood.* 2009;114(21):4687, *Blood.* 2010;115(1):21, *Lancet.* 2004;363(9424):1869, *Cancer Treat Rev.* 2006;32(5):365, *Cancer Treat Rev.* 2011;37(1):3).

CASE 54

A 34-year-old male is referred by his primary care physician for further evaluation of weakness, fatigue, and easy bruising. Physical examination reveals petechial rash. Laboratory workup shows leukocyte count 68,200/μL, hemoglobin 9.7 g/dL, and platelet count 6,000/μL. Coagulation parameters show mild prolongation of PT and PTT at 17 and 46 seconds, respectively. Flow cytometry reveals increased population of cells expressing CD13 and CD33, with negative expression of CD34 and HLA-DR. Myeloperoxidase staining is positive. Testing for nonspecific esterase is negative. Peripheral smear is shown below.

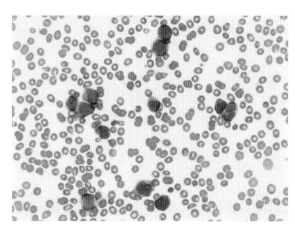

CASE FIGURE 54-1

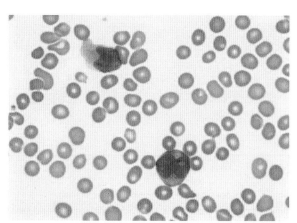

CASE FIGURE 54-2

QUESTION 1

★ What is the most likely diagnosis?

A. Acute promyelocytic leukemia (APL)
B. Acute monocytic leukemia
C. Acute lymphoblastic leukemia
D. Burkitt leukemia
E. Chronic myeloid leukemia

Answer: A. Peripheral slide reveals blasts with bilobed "butterfly" nuclei and sparse or no cytoplasmic granules, which should raise suspicion for the microgranular variant of APL. Fluorescence in situ hybridization (FISH) for t(15;17) confirmed a diagnosis of APL. Negative staining for nonspecific esterase rules out a monocytic differentiation of these blasts. The clinical presentation with leukocytosis, coagulopathy, lack of CD34 and HLA-DR expression, and positivity for myeloperoxidase is characteristic of microgranular APL. This variant of APL constitutes 25% of APL cases, usually presents with leukocytosis, and is associated with a higher risk of coagulopathy, and can be confused with AML of monocytic origin; however, expression of myeloperoxidase and lack of staining for nonspecific esterase provide a useful differentiating tool (*Br J Haematol.* 1982;50(2):201, *Blood.* 1998;91(9):3093).

CASE 55

A 2-week old infant is referred for further evaluation after workup revealed leukocyte count of 120,000/μL, hemoglobin 7.2 g/dL, and platelet count 8,000/μL. Flow cytometry reveals increased expression of CD13, CD19, CD20, and CD33. Peripheral blood smear is shown.

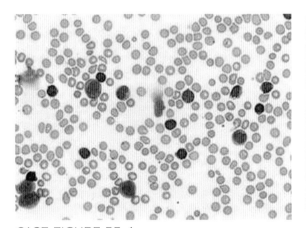

CASE FIGURE 55-1

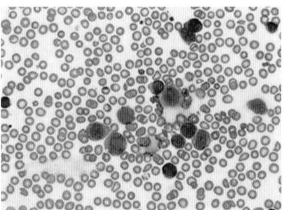

CASE FIGURE 55-2

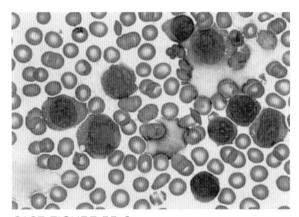

CASE FIGURE 55-3

QUESTION 1

☆ What is the most likely diagnosis?

A. Chronic myeloid leukemia (CML)
B. Chronic lymphocytic leukemia (CLL)
C. Mixed phenotype acute leukemia (MPAL)
D. Acute myeloid leukemia (AML)
E. Acute lymphoblastic leukemia (ALL)

Answer: C. Peripheral slide reveals the presence of two populations of blasts: one with large cells with high nuclear to cytoplasmic ratio, dispersed chromatin, and prominent nucleoli, and another population with small cells with nucleoli and less dispersed chromatin. Flow cytometry reveals expression of both myeloid and lymphoid markers. This is characteristic of MPAL, a condition that comprises less than 5% of acute leukemia cases and is usually associated with a poor prognosis (*Leukemia.* 2010;24(11):1844, *Leukemia.* 2010;24(7):1392, *Blood.* 2011;117(11):3163).

QUESTION 2

☆ What is the most common cytogenetic abnormality in MPAL?

A. t(9;22)
B. 11q23 translocation
C. t(4;11)
D. Complex karyotype
E. t(8;14)

Answer: A. Philadelphia chromosome was detected in 20% of cases of MPAL. Translocations involving the mixed lineage leukemia gene (*MLL*) at 11q23 are seen in 8% of cases (*Blood.* 2011;117(11):3163).

CASE 56

A 59-year-old female with prior history of breast cancer treated adjuvantly with doxorubicin, cyclophosphamide, and docetaxel 3 years previously presents for further evaluation of fatigue. Patient reports that she had a normal physical examination and laboratory workup during her yearly follow-up with her primary care physician 6 months previously. Physical examination reveals pallor and petechial rash with no lymphadenopathy or hepatosplenomegaly. Laboratory workup shows leukocyte count of 133,700/μL, hemoglobin 7.2 g/dL, and platelet count of 8,000/μL. Flow cytometry reveals predominance of CD13, CD33, and CD34 expression. Peripheral slide is shown below.

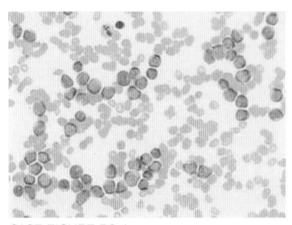

CASE FIGURE 56-1

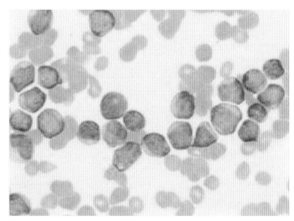

CASE FIGURE 56-2

QUESTION 1

✭ What is the most likely diagnosis?

A. Acute myeloid leukemia (AML)
B. Chronic myeloid leukemia (CML)
C. Myelophthisic anemia (MA)
D. Acute lymphoblastic leukemia (ALL)
E. Myelofibrosis (MF)

Answer: A. Peripheral blood smear demonstrates leukocytes with high nuclear-to-cytoplasmic ratio, dispersed chromatin, and prominent nucleoli. This picture in addition to extreme leukocytosis and bicytopenia is most consistent with AML, specifically therapy related AML (t-AML). There is no evidence of the typical "myeloid left shift" seen in CML cases and there is no evidence of tear drop red blood cell forms or hepatosplenomegaly as would be expected in MF. Bone marrow involvement by recurrent metastatic breast cancer causing MA might result in a leukoerythroblastic picture in peripheral blood that is not seen in this case. Flow cytometry results reveal increased expression of myeloid markers, and thus do not support the diagnosis of ALL.

QUESTION 2

✵ What is the most likely cytogenetic abnormality expected in this case?

A. −5
B. t(9;11)
C. −7
D. t(15;17)
E. t(9;22)

Answer: B. t-AML presenting within the first 3 years after treatment with a topoisomerase II inhibitor (doxorubicin), and with no antecedent myelodysplastic syndrome, is most consistent with t-AML following topoisomerase II inhibitor use. The most common associated cytogenetic abnormality involves the *MLL* gene at chromosome 11q23, and t(9;11) is the most commonly reported chromosomal abnormality. Prior exposure to radiation or alkylating agents results in t-AML that has a longer latency (5 to 7 years), is usually preceded by MDS, and is characterized by complex or monosomal karyotype (−5 or −7). Regardless of previous therapy, t-AML is associated with worse outcomes compared with de novo cases (*Br J Haematol.* 2000;109(1):13, *Semin Oncol.* 2008;35(4):418, *Blood.* 2003;102(1):43).

CASE 57

A 83-year-old female presents for evaluation of fatigue. Physical examination reveals no hepatosplenomegaly or lymphadenopathy. Laboratory workup shows leukocyte count 187,000/μL, hemoglobin 7.3 g/dL, and platelet count 14,000/μL. Flow cytometry reveals an increased number of cells expressing CD13 and CD33. Approximately 10% to 15% of leukocytes stained positive for myeloperoxidase (MPO). Peripheral smear is shown below.

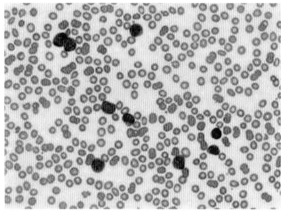

CASE FIGURE 57-1

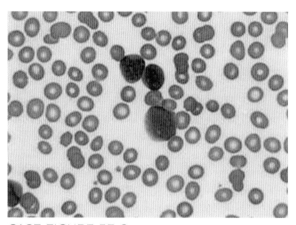

CASE FIGURE 57-2

QUESTION 1

⋆ What is the most likely diagnosis?

A. Acute lymphoblastic leukemia (ALL)
B. Acute myeloid leukemia with minimal differentiation
C. Acute myeloid leukemia without maturation
D. Chronic myelomonocytic leukemia (CMML)
E. Chronic myeloid leukemia (CML)

Answer: C. Peripheral smear shows the presence of blasts which appear to bear features of both myeloid and lymphoid lineages. Flow cytometry results support the diagnosis of AML, given the expression of myeloid markers. MPO stain is positive, which also helps confirm the myeloid lineage of these blasts. Flow cytometry and MPO staining serve as quick gross diagnostic tools to differentiate AML from ALL. Positivity for MPO in at least 3% of leukocytes diagnoses AML without maturation, as cases of AML with minimal differentiation stain negative for MPO.

A 55-year-old male with history of heavy alcohol use is admitted to the hospital secondary to severe alcohol intoxication. Physical examination reveals jaundice and tender hepatomegaly. Laboratory workup shows leukocyte count 25,700/μL, hemoglobin 7.7 g/dL, mean corpuscular volume (MCV) 103 fL, and platelet count 277,000/μL. Total bilirubin level is 24.5 mg/dL with a direct component of 21.7 mg/dL, AST 229 U/L, ALT 85 U/L, and PT 18.6 seconds. Vitamin B_{12} and folate are normal, while ferritin is elevated at 6,000 ng/mL. Peripheral blood smear and iron staining of peripheral blood smear are shown below.

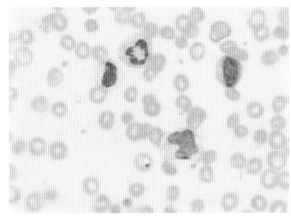

CASE FIGURE 58-1

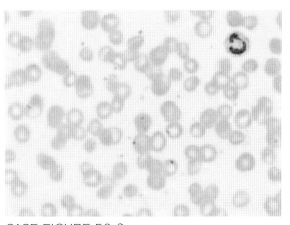

CASE FIGURE 58-2

CASE FIGURE 58-3

QUESTION 1

✷ What is the most likely etiology of his anemia?

A. Spur cell anemia (SCA)
B. Autoimmune hemolytic anemia (AIHA)
C. Acquired sideroblastic anemia (SA)
D. Aplastic anemia (AA)
E. Anemia of chronic disease (ACD)

Answer: C. Peripheral blood smear reveals small inclusions in the red blood cells that stain positive with Prussian blue for iron. These inclusions are called Pappenheimer bodies and represent lysomome containing iron–protein complexes. Such red cells are siderocytes. Siderocytes are considered to be the peripheral blood counterparts of bone marrow sideroblasts and are seen in cases of acquired SA secondary to heavy alcohol use. These cases are characterized by increased iron stores. Abstinence from alcohol is associated with disappearance of siderocytes and improvement in anemia. SCA is associated with severe liver disease; however, this case does not exhibit increased acanthocytes, and there is no evidence of clinically significant hemolysis, no reticulocytosis, or indirect hyperbilirubinemia as would be expected in cases of SCA or AIHA. Normal platelet count and leukocytosis are not consistent with the diagnosis of AA. Other conditions that are contributory to the development of anemia in heavy alcohol users include the presence of hypersplenism, chronic gastrointestinal bleeding, direct cytotoxic effect of alcohol on the bone marrow, nutritional deficiencies, and anemia of chronic disease (*Medicine Baltimore.* 1986;65(5):322, *Hematol Oncol Clin North Am.* 1987;1(2):321).

A 8-year-old boy with history of recurrent cutaneous Staphylococcal infections from infancy is referred for further evaluation secondary to an abnormal reported peripheral blood smear review during a recent hospital admission. There is no preceding history of bleeding. Physical examination reveals silver colored hair and mild splenomegaly with no lymphadenopathy. Laboratory workup shows leukocyte count of 6,700/μL, hemoglobin 12.3 g/dL, and platelet count 376,000/μL. Peripheral blood smear is shown below.

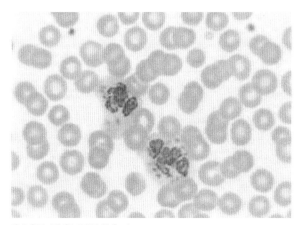

CASE FIGURE 59-1

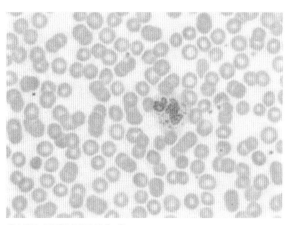

CASE FIGURE 59-2

QUESTION 1

⭐ What is the most likely diagnosis?

A. May–Hegglin anomaly (MHA)
B. Chediak–Higashi syndrome (CHS)
C. Chronic granulomatous disease (CGD)
D. Myeloperoxidase deficiency (MPO deficiency)
E. Leukocyte adhesion defect (LAD)

Answer: B. Peripheral blood smear reveals the presence of giant azurophilic granules in neutrophils. The combination of recurrent pyogenic infections from young age, gray–silver hair discoloration, and the presence of giant azurophilic granules is most consistent with the diagnosis of CHS. CHS is an autosomal recessive disorder and patients with CHS usually present during infancy or early childhood with recurrent pyogenic infections and oculocutaneous albinism. Neutropenia is common, and some cases may manifest mild degrees of bleeding tendency. Of interest a similar disorder occurs in mink, who are inbred for their unusual color (silver–gray), but usually expire by 1 year of age. May–Hegglin anomaly usually presents with giant platelets, thrombocytopenia and less dramatic neutrophil inclusions, with no increased incidence of infections. The presentation described is not typical of CGD, MPO deficiency or LAD (*Curr Opin Hematol.* 2008;15(1):22, *Blood.* 1976;47(6):941, *Br J Haematol.* 1985;59(3):471).

QUESTION 2

Patient is treated conservatively and followed up for the next 2 years till he presents to the emergency department complaining of persistent fever, left-sided abdominal pain, and increased bruising. Patient also reports increased frequency of infections over the preceding 2 months. Physical examination reveals diffuse lymphadenopathy with worsening splenomegaly and new-onset moderate pancytopenia.

☆ What is the most likely explanation of his presentation?

A. Septic shock
B. Hemophagocytic lymphohistiocytosis (HLH)
C. Transformation to acute myeloid leukemia (AML)
D. Progression to myelofibrosis (MF)
E. Transformation to small lymphocytic lymphoma (SLL)

Answer: B. The accelerated phase of CHS resembles a HLH syndrome and is usually a terminal event, eventually affecting the majority of cases. It presents with massive lymphohistiocytic organ infiltration, worsening immune dysfunction and pancytopenia, increased bleeding tendency with hepatosplenomegaly, and lymphadenopathy. It is thought to be precipitated by an infection with Epstein–Barr virus (EBV) that in the setting of an abnormal immune surveillance and inflammatory milieu predisposes to uncontrolled lymphoproliferation (*Cancer.* 1958;56(3):524, *J Clin Immunol.* 1986;6(4):299).

QUESTION 3

☆ What is the underlying genetic defect in CHS?

A. Mutation in *LYST* gene
B. Mutation in *ELA2* gene
C. Mutation in *SBDS* gene
D. Mutation in *DKC1* gene
E. Mutation in *DBA* gene

Answer: A. The underlying defect in CHS is a mutation in lysosomal trafficking regulator gene (*LYST*), located on chromosome 1q, which results in defective organellar protein trafficking and lysosomal function. Mutations in *ELA2* are associated with cyclic neutropenia and severe congenital neutropenia, while mutations in *SBDS* are associated with Shwachman–Diamond syndrome. Dyskeratosis congenita and Diamond–Blackfan anemia are associated with mutations in *DKC1* and *DBA*, respectively (*Nature.* 1996;382(6588):262, *Nat Genet.* 1996;14(3):307).

A 56-year-old female with no significant medical history is admitted to the hospital with an acute left subdural hematoma after a fall. Physical examination is significant for normal mental status, diffuse ecchymoses, and massive splenomegaly. Patient denies preceding abdominal pain, weight loss, fevers, or night sweats. Laboratory evaluation shows leukocyte count of 119,000/μL, hemoglobin 8 g/dL, and platelet count 102,000/μL. Eosinophil and basophil counts are normal. Peripheral slide is shown below.

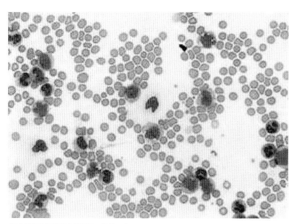

CASE FIGURE 60-1

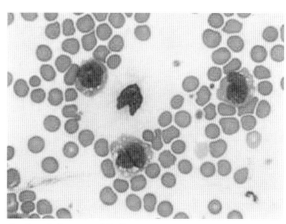

CASE FIGURE 60-2

QUESTION 1

✰ What is the most likely diagnosis based on the available clinical information?

A. Chronic myeloid leukemia (CML)
B. Acute myeloid leukemia (AML)
C. Chronic myelomonocytic leukemia (CMML)
D. Myelofibrosis (MF)
E. Chronic lymphocytic leukemia (CLL)

Answer: C. Peripheral slide reveals monocytosis with absence of basophilia or eosinophilia. The main differential diagnoses in this case are CMML and CML. The absence of eosinophilia, and especially basophilia, and no left shift in myeloid cells, argue against the diagnosis of CML. There is no evidence of myeloid blasts in the peripheral blood to support the diagnosis of AML, and there is no evidence of lymphocytosis as would be expected in CLL. Testing for *BCR-ABL* translocation is essential in distinguishing between CMML and CML, as CMML would be expected to test negative. CMML is classified as an overlap entity exhibiting features of both myelodysplastic and myeloproliferative syndromes in addition to a persistently elevated monocyte count in excess of 1,000/μL. It presents with monocytosis in addition to anemia, thrombocytopenia, dysfunctional platelets, and splenomegaly (*Leukemia.* 2008;22(7):1308, *Leuk Lymphoma.* 2008;49(7):1292, *J Neurosci Rural Pract.* 2012;3(1):98, *Br J Haematol.* 2011;153(2):149).

QUESTION 2

✴ Bone marrow biopsy was obtained and revealed hypercellularity with increased number of myeloid blasts at 15%. What is the final diagnosis?

A. Chronic myelomonocytic leukemia type 1 (CMML-1)
B. Chronic myelomonocytic leukemia type 2 (CMML-2)
C. Acute myeloid leukemia (AML)

Answer: B. Presence of 10% to 19% bone marrow blasts supports the diagnosis of CMML-2. Cases of CMML-1 are diagnosed when bone marrow blast count if less than 10%, while bone marrow blast count in excess of 20% is diagnostic of AML (*Br J Haematol.* 2011;153(2):149).

A 53-year-old male presents with confusion, progressive weakness, and weight loss. Physical examination reveals bilateral inguinal lymphadenopathy and splenomegaly. Laboratory workup is significant for a leukocyte count of 94,000/μL, hemoglobin of 7.4 g/dL, and platelet count of 27,000/μL. Creatinine is elevated at 5.7 mg/dL, with no prior history of renal impairment. LDH and uric acid levels are found to be elevated at 1,850 U/L and 13.8 mg/dL, respectively. CT scan of the abdomen reveals massive lymphadenopathy. Flow cytometry of the peripheral blood shows expression of CD19, CD20, and HLA-DR on the surface of the abnormal leukocytes. Peripheral blood smear is shown below.

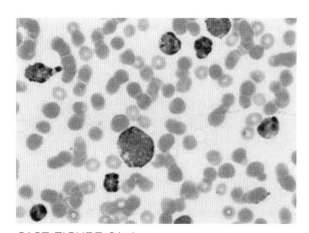

CASE FIGURE 61-1

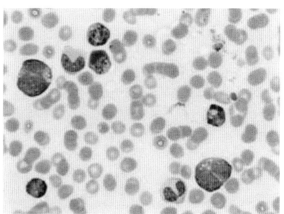

CASE FIGURE 61-2

QUESTION 1

✯ What is the most likely diagnosis?

A. Chronic lymphocytic leukemia (CLL)
B. Intravascular large cell lymphoma (ILCL)
C. Diffuse large B-cell lymphoma (DLBCL)
D. Adult T-cell leukemia/lymphoma (ATLL)
E. Sezary syndrome (SS)

Answer: C. Peripheral slide reveals evidence of circulating large leukocytes exhibiting prominent nucleoli and typical B-cell markers. Imaging studies revealed massive lymph node conglomerate in the abdomen. DLBCL presenting in leukemic phase is the most appropriate of the choices given. Lymph node biopsy confirmed the diagnosis of DLBCL. Lack of expression of T-cell markers excludes the diagnosis of ATLL and SS, both of which are T-cell malignancies. CLL is excluded by the lack of typical morphology and negative expression of CD5 and CD23. ILCL is a rare subtype of large cell lymphoma, most commonly of B-cell lineage, that is characterized by the proliferation of lymphoma cell within small blood vessels with absence of circulating lymphoma cells and lack of extravascular tumor masses (*Br J Haematol.* 2012;158(5):608, *J Clin Oncol.* 2007;25(21):3168, *Blood.* 2007;109(2):478, *Br J Haematol.* 2004;127(2):173).

QUESTION 2

✶ Of the options listed, what is the most common site of extranodal involvement?

A. Spleen
B. Lung
C. Liver
D. Bone
E. Cerebrospinal spinal fluid (CSF)

Answer: A. Extranodal involvement is seen in all cases of DLBCL presenting in leukemic phase. According to one study, bone marrow involvement was present in 100% of cases, followed by spleen (62%), lung (41%), liver (21%), bone (17%), CSF (14%), and bowel (7%). This is in contrast with ILCL, where extranodal involvement is much less commonly observed (*Br J Haematol.* 2012;158(5):608, *J Clin Oncol.* 2007;25(21):3168, *Blood.* 2007;109(2):478, *Br J Haematol.* 2004;127(2):173).

CASE 62

A 32-year-old male presents for evaluation of skin lesions, increased bruising, and fatigue. Examination reveals a conglomerate of nodular skin lesions involving the skin of the face and upper trunk. There is no hepatosplenomegaly or lymphadenopathy. Diffuse petechial rash is seen over both lower extremities. Laboratory evaluation reveals leukocyte count of 57,200/μL, hemoglobin of 7.8 g/dL, and platelet count of 8,000/μL. Flow cytometry reveals expression of CD11c, CD13, CD14, CD33, CD34, CD68, and HLA-DR. Staining for myeloperoxidase (MPO) and nonspecific esterase (NSE) shows positivity in 40% and 45%, respectively. Peripheral blood smear is shown below.

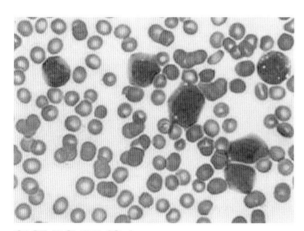

CASE FIGURE 62-1

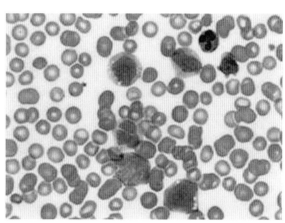

CASE FIGURE 62-2

QUESTION 1

★ What is the most likely diagnosis?

A. Acute myeloid leukemia with maturation
B. Acute myelomonocytic leukemia (AMML)
C. Acute megakaryoblastic leukemia (AMKL)
D. Acute myeloid leukemia with minimal differentiation
E. Acute promyelocytic leukemia (APL)

Answer: B. Peripheral slide reveals the presence of myeloid blast cells exhibiting dispersed chromatin and high nuclear-to-cytoplasmic ratio. The blasts appear to bear morphologic resemblance to monocytes and express monocytic cell surface markers: CD11c, CD14, and CD68. Positive staining for MPO and NSE, in addition to the characteristic skin involvement, is most consistent with AMML. Cutaneous involvement can be seen in 15% of AML cases and is most characteristic of AML with monocytic or myelomonocytic differentiation, where it has been reported in up to 50% of cases. Positivity for MPO excludes AML with minimal differentiation because, by definition, these cases are negative for MPO. Monocytic markers are usually absent in cases of AML with maturation. Flow cytometry in cases of APL is characteristically negative for CD34 and HLA-DR (*Blood.* 2011;118(14):3785, *Ann Hematol.* 2002;81(2):90, *Blood.* 1980;55(1):71, *Blood.* 2011;118(14):3785).

CASE 63

A 30-year-old female patient is seen for evaluation of fatigue. Initial labs show a hemoglobin of 7.6 g/dL, MCV of 106 fL, WBC of 3,200/μL, and platelets of 178,000/μL. LDH is 1,200 U/L and haptoglobin is low. On review of symptoms, she states that her urine is dark in the morning, but clears toward the evening. Test tubes showing serial urine samples are shown below.

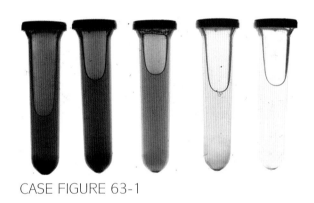

CASE FIGURE 63-1

QUESTION 1

☆ Which of the following tests would most likely lead to a definitive diagnosis in this patient?

A. Cytogenetic analysis of a bone marrow aspirate
B. Direct antigen test
C. Flow cytometry of peripheral blood
D. Complement levels
E. Urine protein electrophoresis

Answer: C. The urine demonstrates early morning hemoglobinuria, which clears during the day. This observation in a patient with evidence of hemolysis (increased LDH and decreased haptoglobin) should raise concern for paroxysmal nocturnal hemoglobinuria (PNH). Hemolytic anemia in PNH is due to increased sensitivity to complement lysis secondary to deficiency of CD55 (decay accelerating factor) and CD 59 (membrane inhibitor of reactive lysis). Flow cytometry can detect decreased expression of these complement proteins and is a standard test used in the diagnosis of PNH.

QUESTION 2

✲ PNH is not associated with which of the following conditions?

A. Development of aplastic anemia
B. Evolution to acute myeloid leukemia
C. Severe IgG deficiency
D. Spontaneous thrombosis of the portal vein
E. Hemorrhage due to severe thrombocytopenia

Answer: C. PNH is associated with both evolution to aplastic anemia (AA) and, in some cases, development of acute myeloid leukemia (AML) in 1% to 2% of cases. Patients with PNH are at increased risk of both venous thrombosis and hemorrhage. PNH is not associated with immunoglobulin deficiency.

QUESTION 3

✲ Which of the following is the most common pathophysiologic mechanism in PNH?

A. Mutation in the PIG-A gene
B. Deficiency of ADAMTS-13
C. IgM antibodies to the I antigen on red blood cells
D. Donath–Landsteiner antibodies
E. Acquired complement deficiency

Answer: A. PNH is an acquired hematopoietic stem cell disorder that results from somatic mutation of the PIG-A gene. The protein encoded by PIG-A gene is needed for the synthesis of glycosyl phosphatidylinositol (GPI) that serves as a membrane anchor for cellular proteins. Due to the mutant PIG-A, there is a deficiency of CD55 and CD59, and thus peripheral blood erythrocytes derived from the abnormal clone lack the ability to restrict cell surface activation of the alternate complement pathway, which results in hemolytic anemia.

QUESTION 4

✲ The patient is treated with red blood cell infusions, folic acid supplementation, iron supplementation, and oral glucocorticoids and is well for several months with an improvement in anemia and fatigue. At one year, the patient shows worsening anemia and fatigue and is diagnosed with portal vein thrombosis; she is started on oral anticoagulation. Which of the choices is the next appropriate step in management?

A. Immunosuppressive therapy with azathioprine
B. Chemotherapy with cyclophosphamide and high-dose steroids
C. Immunotherapy with rituximab
D. Evaluation for bone marrow transplantation
E. Weekly plasma exchange

Answer: D. Allogeneic stem cell transplantation (SCT) with an HLA-matched donor should be offered, since this is the only curative option. However, SCT may be associated with serious complications, including graft-versus-host disease, infection, and death, and thus should be reserved for patients who have failed eculizumab. Plasma exchange, immunosuppression, chemotherapy, and rituximab are not standard options in the treatment of PNH.

QUESTION 5

✶   She was started on eculizumab. What is the mechanism of action of this agent?

A. Anti-CD52 antibody
B. Anticomplement protein C5
C. Inhibits production of multiple opsonization molecules
D. Allosteric inhibition of T-cell antigen receptors

Answer: B. Eculizumab is a humanized monoclonal antibody that binds to C5, preventing its activation to C5b, and hence inhibiting the formation of the membrane attack complex. Treatment with eculizumab ameliorates hemolytic anemia and decreases transfusion requirements and thromboembolic events. It is not beneficial in patients who have bone marrow failure. Alemtuzumab is a monoclonal antibody against CD52 that has been used in the treatment of lymphoproliferative disorders.

QUESTION 6

✶   Which of the following is a serious potential adverse effect of eculizumab?

A. Hepatic failure
B. Pericardial effusion leading to tamponade
C. Meningococcal infection
D. Reactivation of latent hepatitis B
E. Acute closed-angle glaucoma

Answer: C. Eculizumab binds to C5 and blocks the terminal complement sequence. Patients lacking the terminal complement proteins, C5 to C9, are at risk for Neisseria infections. Vaccination against Neisseria meningitides is recommended prior to therapy with this agent.

CASE 64

A 79-year-old Caucasian man presents with a chief complaint of back pain. Hemoglobin is 9.7 g/dL, leukocyte count 7,600/μL, and platelet count 214,000/μL. BUN is 26 mg/dL, creatinine 2.1 mg/dL, total protein 9.0 g/dL, albumin 3.1 g/dL, and calcium 10.9 mg/dL. The images below show the bone marrow aspirate and a skull film from the skeletal survey.

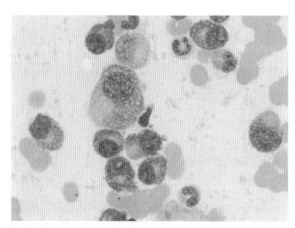

CASE FIGURE 64-1

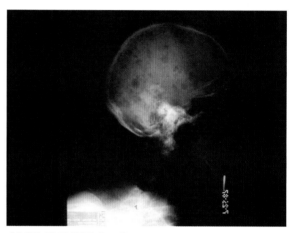

CASE FIGURE 64-2

QUESTION 1

☆ Which of the following lab tests is necessary to complete the staging of the patient according to the International Staging System (ISS)?

A. Serum M-protein level
B. Sedimentation rate
C. Assay for urine light chains
D. Beta-2 microglobulin
E. Quantitative free light chain assay

Answer: D. The bone marrow aspirate shows increased cells with blue cytoplasm, a perinuclear hof, and an eccentric nucleus with clumped chromatin, characteristic of plasma cells. Skull radiograph depicts the punched out lesions typical of multiple myeloma (MM). The ISS uses albumin and beta-2 microglobulin levels to stratify patients with MM into one of three levels.

QUESTION 2

✷ Further evaluation reveals a beta-2 microglobulin level of 4.7 mg/L, free light chain assay showing increased kappa/lambda ratio of 7.9, and the bone marrow aspirate noted 13% plasma cells. To establish a diagnosis of MM, what is the most pertinent finding?

A. Evidence of end-organ damage
B. Percent plasma cells
C. Beta-2 microglobulin level
D. K:L ratio

Answer: A. Regardless of the percentage of bone marrow plasma cells or the level of beta-2 micro-globulin or free light chains, the presence of end-organ damage in the form hypercalcemia, renal insufficiency, anemia, or bone lesions (CRAB) is necessary to establish a diagnosis of MM.

QUESTION 3

✷ What chromosome abnormality is not commonly found in patients with MM?

A. t(11;14)(q13;q32)
B. 13q14 deletion
C. t(4;14)(p16;q32)
D. Trisomy 12
E. 17p13 deletion

Answer: D. Cytogenetic abnormalities have been detected by FISH in 80% or more of patients with MM. Deletion 13q is the most common abnormality, reported in 40% to 50% of newly diagnosed patients using FISH. The prevalence of t(11;14) is 15% to 20%; t(4;14) is 15%; and 17p deletion is 5% to 10%. Trisomy 12 has been reported in association with lymphomas and chronic lymphocytic leukemia.

QUESTION 4

✷ Which of the following options reflects the correct *descending* order for the type of immuno-globulin that is responsible for the M-spike in MM?

A. IgG, IgD, IgA
B. IgG, IgA, IgD
C. IgD, IgG, IgA
D. They occur with equal frequency

Answer: B. The serum M-protein is IgG in 53%, IgA in 25%, and IgD in 1% of patients.

QUESTION 5

✶ Which of the following treatment regimens would not be appropriate for a patient who is considered a candidate for bone marrow transplantation?

A. Melphalan-prednisone-lenalidomide
B. Bortezomib-lenalidomide-dexamethasone
C. Lenalidomide-dexamethasone
D. Thalidomide-dexamethasone

Answer: A. Alkylating agents, such as melphalan, are not recommended in patients who are transplant-eligible because these agents damage hematopoietic stem cells and interfere with adequate stem cell mobilization.

QUESTION 6

✶ The patient is treated with bortezomib-dexamethasone and has a good response, with decrease in serum M-protein, decrease in beta-2 microglobulin, and normalization of creatinine. After 6 months of observation, he is hospitalized with a painful compression fracture, and the M-protein is increased as well as creatinine and serum calcium levels. Therapy is initiated with thalidomide and dexamethasone. What clinical options should be included in his plan of management?

A. Monthly intraocular pressure measurements
B. Serial EKGs
C. Thromboembolism prophylaxis
D. Regular audiologic testing
E. Weekly urinalysis for proteinuria

Answer: C. Thalidomide use in MM is associated with an increased risk of thrombosis, and the risk is increased when thalidomide is combined with dexamethasone and/or chemotherapy. Indeed, thromboembolism is a black box warning with this drug. Patients undergoing thalidomide-based regimens should receive some type of prophylactic anticoagulation, unless there is a contraindication.

QUESTION 7

✶ In determining eligibility for hematopoietic stem cell transplantation in a patient with MM, which of the following would be considered a possible reason for exclusion from transplant?

A. ECOG performance status 2
B. Serum creatinine of 4 mg/dL, not on dialysis
C. Age > 65
D. History of ischemic stoke
E. Failed > 2 lines of treatment

Answer: B. NYHA stage III/IV heart failure, direct bilirubin > 2.0 mg/dL, ECOG PS 3 or 4, age more than 77 years, and serum creatinine > 2.5 unless the patient is established on dialysis are common exclusion criteria used when evaluating patients for HSCT.

A 23-year-old female patient presents with complaints of "spots on my legs." She has been in her normal state of health recently with the exception of cold symptoms that lasted for 5 days and have now resolved. Complete blood count shows hemoglobin of 14.5g/dL, leukocyte count of 8,900/μL, and platelet count of 13,000/μL. Photographs of the patient and her peripheral blood smear are shown below.

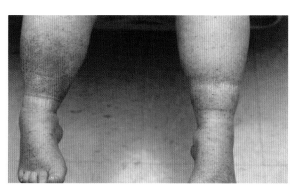

CASE FIGURE 65-1

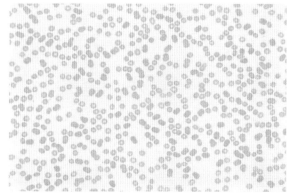

CASE FIGURE 65-2

QUESTION 1

☆ What test(s) would be appropriate in the evaluation of this patient?

A. Bone marrow biopsy and aspiration
B. LDH, haptoglobin, unconjugated bilirubin
C. HIV, hepatitis C, ANA
D. Antiplatelet antibodies
E. ADAMTS-13 level

Answer: C. Blood smear shows an absence of platelets with normal red blood cells. Primary immune thrombocytopenia (ITP) is diagnosed after exclusion of secondary conditions such as HIV infection, hepatitis C, and SLE. Antiplatelet antibodies are not helpful and are not indicated in the evaluation of ITP. ADAMTS-13 deficiency is associated with thrombotic thrombocytopenic purpura (TTP) but the hemoglobin is normal and there are no schistocytes in the blood smear. Bone marrow biopsy is appropriate in older patients to rule out myelodysplastic syndrome (MDS).

QUESTION 2

✷ The patient has hemoglobin level of 14.5 g/dL, platelet count of 13,000/μL, and leukocyte count of 8,900/μL. Which of the treatments below is a reasonable first treatment option in the absence of bleeding symptoms?

A. Plasma exchange
B. Splenectomy
C. Cyclophosphamide
D. Prednisone
E. Rituximab

Answer: D. In patients diagnosed with immune thrombocytopenia, prednisone 1 mg/kg daily is a reasonable choice for first-line therapy in the absence of bleeding symptoms. Plasma exchange does not have a role in treatment of ITP, unlike its primary role in the treatment of TTP. Splenectomy, chemotherapy, and rituximab are all second-line therapies reserved for patients unresponsive to steroid therapy.

QUESTION 3

✷ The peripheral blood smear in a patient with immune thrombocytopenia would most likely demonstrate which of the following abnormal findings?

A. Rouleaux formation
B. Large platelets
C. Schistocytes
D. Howell–Jolly bodies
E. Nucleated red blood cells

Answer: B. The peripheral smear of a patient with ITP may show large platelets, consistent with a bone marrow response of accelerated platelet release. Rouleaux is seen commonly in multiple myeloma, schistocytes in TTP and Howell–Jolly bodies in splenectomized patients or those with hemolytic or megaloblastic anemia, and nucleated red blood cells in conditions of hemolysis or marrow replacement.

CASE 66

A 18-year-old female patient of Iranian descent presents to the emergency room with back and leg pain. Laboratory results reveal leukocyte count of 17,400/μL, hemoglobin of 11.5 g/dL, MCV of 65 fL, and platelet count of 297,000/μL. Peripheral smear is shown below.

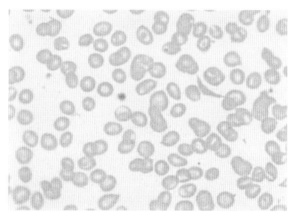

CASE FIGURE 66-1

QUESTION 1

✶ Which of the following choices represents the expected pattern on hemoglobin electrophoresis for this condition?

A. HbS 90%   HbF 8%   HbA2 <3.5%
B. HbC 50%   HbS 45%   HbF 2.5%   HbA2 2.5%
C. HbA 60%   HbS 35%   HbF <2%   HbA2 < 3.5%
D. HbS 60%   HbA 30%   HbF 3%   HbA2 7%

Answer: D. Choice A represents sickle cell disease (SS), choice B represents sickle-HbC disease (SC), choice C represents sickle-cell trait, and choice D represents sickle-beta(+) thalassemia. The peripheral smear shows target cells, which are commonly seen in thalassemia, and a typical drepanocyte (sickle cell). HbC is seen in patients of African descent, whereas thalassemias are associated with Mediterranean populations. In addition, an MCV of 65 µL favors sickle-beta thalassemia. In sickle cell anemia and trait, the MCV is normal, and in SC disease, the MCV may be normal or mildly microcytic.

QUESTION 2

⭐ The clinical severity of sickle-beta(+) thalassemia depends mostly on which of the following?

A. Level of HbA, which varies based on the type of mutation in beta globin chain
B. Level of HbF, which varies based on the specific sickle-cell mutation phenotype
C. Level of HbA2, which is dependent on the type of mutation in alpha chain
D. Level of HbS, which varies based on the specific sickle-cell mutation phenotype

Answer: A. The level of HbA determines the disease severity in patients with sickle-beta(+) thalassemia; the higher the level of Hgb A, the milder the disease (*Br J Haematol.* 1991;77(3):386–91).

QUESTION 3

⭐ The patient improves with vigorous hydration, morphine delivered via PCA, and treatment of bronchitis. Review of her chart shows that she has been admitted to the hospital through the ER with pain crisis 5 times in the last 11 months. The consulting hematologist recommends beginning treatment with hydroxyurea. Although not as well established in the treatment of sickle-beta (+) thalassemia patients, hydroxyurea is known to benefit sickle cell patients through which of the following mechanisms?

A. Increase in HbF
B. Increase in HbA
C. Increase in normal beta-globin chains
D. Decrease in HbS

Answer: A. The clinical benefit from hydroxyurea is primarily through increased fetal hemoglobin levels although effects on RBC hydration and effects on nitric oxide production, as well as other mechanisms, have been proposed (*New Eng J Med.* 2008;358(13): 1362–1369).

QUESTION 4

⭐ Hydroxyurea should not be used in which of the following populations?

A. Children
B. Patients with autoimmune conditions
C. Women of child-bearing age who are not using birth control
D. Patients with congestive heart failure

Answer: C. Based on animal studies, there is significant concern about possible harm to the developing fetus. Close attention to this issue prior to and throughout treatment with hydroxyurea is recommended (*New Eng J Med.* 2008;358(13): 1362–1369).

CASE 67

A 64-year-old female patient with celiac disease and related dermatitis herpetiformis presents to the emergency room complaining of fatigue and blue finger tips. She has been taking dapsone for approximately 3 months. CBC shows leukocyte count 9,500/μL, hemoglobin 7.5 g/dL, and platelet count 176,000/μL. Laboratory informs you that the patient has "green serum," as shown below.

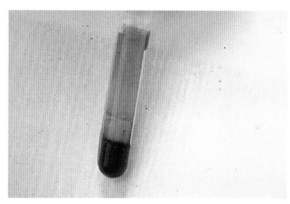

CASE FIGURE 67-1

QUESTION 1

⋆ What is the most likely diagnosis?

A. Carboxyhemoglobinemia
B. Methemoblobinemia
C. Sulfhemoglobinemia

Answer: C. The test tube shows green serum secondary to sulfhemoglobinemia. Sulfhemoglobin is a green-pigmented protein, and is been associated with the use of oxidant medications, occupational exposure to sulfur compounds, air pollution, and recreational drug abuse, and may cause oxidative hemolysis. Unlike for methemoglinemia, methylene blue is not effective for treatment, although most patients with sulfhemoglobinemia are asymptomatic. Methemoglobinemia is associated with choco- late brown blood, and carboxyhemoglobinemia may cause cherry or bright pink nails.

CASE 68

A 57-year-old man presents with fatigue and dyspnea on exertion. Initial laboratory workup shows hemoglobin 10.5 g/dL with an MCV of 85 fL, leukocyte count 11,200/μL, and platelet count 167,000/μL. No lymphadenopathy or splenomegaly was noted on physical exam. Peripheral blood smear is shown below.

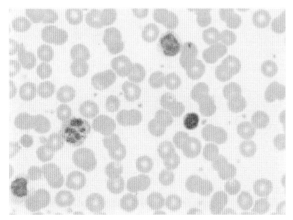

CASE FIGURE 68-1

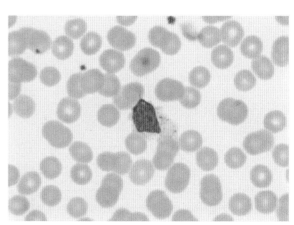

CASE FIGURE 68-2

QUESTION 1

★ Flow cytometry in this patient would typically reveal what results?

A. Positive CD5, CD19, CD20, and CD23
B. Positive for CD3, CD8, and CD57
C. Positive for CD5, CD19, and CD20 but negative for CD23
D. Positive for CD38 and CD138

Answer: B. Peripheral blood smear shows several large granular lymphocytes. T-cell large granular lymphocytic leukemia (T-LGL) is usually positive for the CD markers 3, 8, 16, and 57. Choice A would be consistent with chronic lymphocytic leukemia. Choice C is the immunophenotype of natural killer cell lymphocytosis, and choice D shows markers characteristic of plasma cells. T-cell receptor gene rearrangement was positive in the patient, confirming the diagnostic impression of LGL.

QUESTION 2

✶ What comorbid condition is not found with an increased incidence in patients diagnosed with LGL leukemia?

A. Rheumatoid arthritis (RA)
B. Immune thrombocytopenia
C. Hepatitis C
D. Celiac disease
E. Focal segmental glomerulosclerosis (FSGS)

Answer: E. Both autoimmune conditions (most commonly RA) and infectious diseases (including HIV, hepatitis C, EBV, and CMV) are associated with LGL leukemia. There is no association between FSGS and LGL leukemia. (*Blood.* 2011;117(10): 2764–2774)

QUESTION 3

✶ What is the most common clinical presentation of LGL?

A. Massive splenomegaly and lymphadenopathy
B. Severe anemia requiring transfusion
C. Severe neutropenia and infections
D. Mental status changes secondary to hyperviscosity
E. Purpuric rash secondary to thrombocytopenia

Answer: C. Neutropenia is present in up to 85% of patients with LGL and is commonly severe with an absolute neutrophil count less than 500. Although splenomegaly is seen in 25% to 50% of cases, lymphadenopathy is not common. Severe anemia and thrombocytopenia may occur, but are not as common as leukopenia at presentation. Hyperviscosity is not a clinical feature of LGL leukemia. (*Blood.* 2011;117(10):2764–2774)

QUESTION 4

✶ What best describes the usual clinical course of T-LGL leukemia?

A. Rapid progression with overall survival measured in months
B. Spontaneous regression with recurrence in about one-half of patients
C. Indolent course which often does not require immediate therapy
D. Cure of the disease with successful treatment directed toward an underlying autoimmune condition

Answer: C. The natural history of T-LGL leukemia is one of indolence, with median survival of more than 10 years. Treatment is initiated when cytopenias become significant or associated autoimmune conditions prompt intervention. Spontaneous regression has rarely been described. Although treatment directed toward an underlying autoimmune condition is part of the approach to LGL, control rather than cure is the norm. Recent data suggest that aberrant STAT3 and STAT5b signaling underlie the pathogenesis of this disease. Perhaps treatment with STAT inhibitors may be of benefit (*NEJM.* 2012;366: 1905–1913. *Blood.* 2012;120:3048–3057).

QUESTION 5

★ All of the following choices are appropriate first- or second-line therapy in LGL leukemia except:

A. CHOP chemotherapy
B. Methotrexate
C. Prednisone
D. Cyclophosphamide
E. Cyclosporine

Answer: A. Although there is no gold standard therapy for LGL, immunosuppressive agents, including methotrexate, corticosteroids, cyclophosphamide, and cyclosporine, have been utilized. The most common indication for treatment is recurrent infection. There is no role for CHOP chemotherapy (*Blood.* 2011;117(10):2764–2774).

A 58-year-old man presents with fatigue and weight loss over the past 1 month. On physical exam, he has enlarged lymph nodes and splenomegaly. Hemoglobin is 9.3 g/dL, leukocyte count is 178,000/μL, and platelet count is 85,000/μL. Flow cytometry of the peripheral blood reveals expression of CD5, CD19, and CD 20, and lack of CD23. Cyclin D 1 is positive. The peripheral blood smear is shown below.

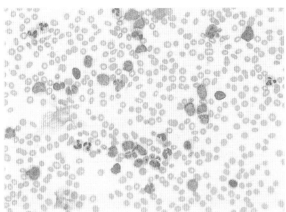

CASE FIGURE 69-1   CASE FIGURE 69-2

QUESTION 1

☆ These findings are most consistent with a diagnosis of:

A. Chronic lymphocytic leukemia
B. Hairy cell leukemia
C. Marginal zone lymphoma
D. Mantle cell lymphoma

Answer: D. The blood smear shows marked leukocytosis with pleomorphic cells with irregular, round, and clefted nuclei with condensed chromatin. This picture, in concert with the immunophenotype, is diagnostic of mantle cell lymphoma (MCL). MCL is typically positive for CD5, CD19, and CD20, but negative for CD23. The typical immunophenotype of CLL is CD5, CD19, CD20, and CD23 positive. Marginal zone lymphoma expresses CD20, but CD5 and CD23 are negative. The morphology is not characteristic of hairy cell leukemia. Mantle cell lymphoma may present in a leukemic phase and portends a poor prognosis with a poor response to chemotherapy (*Cancer.* 1999;86:850–857).

QUESTION 2

✻ What is the most common clinical presentation of mantle cell lymphoma (MCL)?

A. Asymptomatic with abnormal blood counts
B. Advanced disease with lymphadenopathy
C. CNS involvement with meningismus
D. Fever, drenching night sweats, and weight loss

Answer: B. Most patients with MCL lymphoma present at an advanced stage, with lymphadenopathy but without B symptoms. Extradodal involvement makes up about 20% to 25% of cases, including the intestine (often as multiple lymphomatous polyposis) and Waldeyer's ring. CNS involvement is rare (*Blood.* 1997;89:2067–2078).

QUESTION 3

✻ What cytogenetic abnormality is associated with mantle cell lymphoma?

A. t(11;14)
B. t(14;18)
C. (8;21)
D. t(2;5)

Answer: A. t(11;14) is the characteristic genetic alteration in MCL. t(14;18) is associated with follicular lymphoma, t(8;21) with AML, and t(2;5) with anaplastic large cell lymphoma.

A 46-year-old man with a history of non-Hodgkin lymphoma presents with myalgias, fever, and headache. Central nervous symptoms worsened, and he became seriously ill and was admitted to the intensive care unit for evaluation and treatment. Of note, the patient stated he had been working in the woods and thought he may have had a tick bite. He last received treatment for lymphoma 2 years previously. Laboratory shows a leukocyte count of 3,200/μL, hemoglobin 12.3 g/dL, and platelet count 47,000/μL. An image from the peripheral blood smear is shown below.

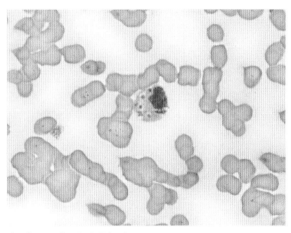

CASE FIGURE 70-1

QUESTION 1

✶ Rickettsial disease is suspected based on the patient's presentation and reported recent tick bites. Which of the following is the most likely diagnosis?

A. Lyme disease
B. Ehrlichiosis/anaplasmosis (HME/HGA)
C. Rocky mountain spotted fever (RMSF)
D. Tularemia

Answer: B. The blood smear shows morulae in the cytoplasm of a leukocyte. This finding plus the patient's presentation of fever, myalgias, headache, leukopenia, and thrombocytopenia is consistent with a diagnosis of ehrlichiosis (human monocytic ehrlichiosis, caused by *Ehrlichia chaffeensis*, or human granulocytic anaplasmosis, caused by *Anaplasma phagocytophilum*). A diagnosis of ehrlichiosis was made in the patient by serology immunofluorescence testing. Morulae are cytoplasmic membrane-bound vacuoles that contain hundreds of gram negative bacteria. Morulae may be detected in the peripheral blood smear in up to 50% to 80% of patients, especially in immunocompromised hosts. Ehrlichiosis is a tick-borne disease, with a clinical spectrum varying from a mild influenza-like illness to a fulminant sepsis syndrome with multiorgan failure. The presentations of these diseases overlap with other rickettsial conditions, but unlike Lyme disease and RMSF, characteristic intracytoplasmic inclusions are frequently found on the peripheral smear in HME/HGA.

QUESTION 2

✮ Which test is not used to confirm the diagnosis of ehrlichiosis/anaplasmosis?

A. Indirect fluorescent antibody testing
B. PCR
C. Cell culture
D. Enzyme-linked immunosorbent assay

Answer: C. Culture of erhlichiae organisms has been rarely successful. The other listed choices are all used to confirm the diagnosis.

QUESTION 3

✮ In terms of differentiating human monocytic erhlichiosis (HME) from human granulocytic anaplasmosis (HGA), which of the following is true?

A. Rash is found in about 30% of patients with HME, but is rare in patients with HGA
B. Liver enzyme elevations are found in 50% of patients with HGA, but in less than 10% of patients with HME
C. Only HGA has been proven to occur in New England
D. Thrombocytopenia occurs in most patients with HME, but only rarely in HGA

Answer: A. Rash is rare in HGA, but occurs in almost one-third of HME cases. There are no differences in the incidence of liver enzyme elevation or thrombocytopenia between HME and HGA. Both conditions have been found to occur in New England.

QUESTION 4

✮ What is the appropriate treatment for HME/HGA infection?

A. Ciprofloxacin, 500 mg BID, for 10 days
B. Erythromycin, 500 mg BID, for 21 days
C. Doxycycline, 100 mg BID, for 10 days
D. Hydroxychloroquine, 400 mg BID, for 21 days

Answer: C. Doxycycline is the recommended treatment and is usually continued for 7 to 10 days.

A 73-year-old man with anemia requiring transfusions for the past 3 months presents for further evaluation. Leukocyte count is 4,900/ μL, hemoglobin 7.9 g/dL, MCV 99 fL, platelet count 176,000/μL, and reticulocyte production index 0.1%. LDH is 182 U/L. On physical exam, he has no hepatosplenomegaly or lymphadenopathy. The peripheral blood smear is shown below.

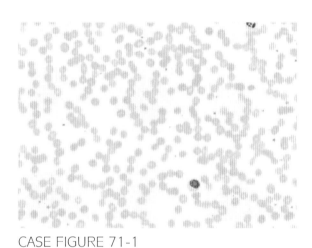

CASE FIGURE 71-1

QUESTION 1

☆ Based on the clinical presentation, lab values, and normal appearance of the peripheral blood smear, pure red cell aplasia (PRCA) is considered. What test would be of limited benefit in the evaluation of suspected PRCA?

A. CT of the chest
B. Flow cytometry of peripheral blood for CD55 and CD59
C. Viral studies including parvovirus
D. Antinuclear antibodies
E. TCR gene rearrangement assay

Answer: B. Flow cytometry showing the absence of CD55 and CD59 would be consistent with a diagnosis of paroxysmal nocturnal hemoglobinuria (PNH). However, such patients usually have hemolytic anemia with reticulocytosis. The other choices are appropriate to evaluate for the presence of thymoma (CT chest), viral infections—especially parvovirus B19—the presence of autoantibodies, and TCR gene rearrangement to detect large granular lymphocytic leukemia. The latter has been reported to be one of the most common causes of PRCA.

QUESTION 2

✴ What statement accurately describes the incidence and response to resection between PRCA and thymoma?

A. The incidence of thymoma in patients with PRCA is near 30%, and resection leads to remission in 70% of patients.
B. The incidence of thymoma in patients with PRCA is near 5%, and resection leads to remission in 70% of patients.
C. The incidence of thymoma in patients with PRCA is 5% to 15%, and resection leads to remission in less than 40% of patients.
D. The incidence of thymoma in patients with PRCA is 5% to 15%, and resection leads to remission in more than 90% of patients.

Answer: C. Although the association between thymoma and PRCA is well recognized, the actual incidence of thymoma as a causative mechanism is low, and modern series suggest that the effect of resection of thymoma on the course of PRCA is not as beneficial as previously thought.

QUESTION 3

✴ First-line therapy for PRCA includes all of the following except:

A. Rituximab
B. Cyclosporine
C. Cyclophosphamide plus corticosteroids
D. Corticosteroids alone

Answer: A. Rituximab is considered for relapsed or resistant disease, along with several other agents, including intravenous immunoglobulin, azathioprine, antithymocyte globulin and alemtuzumab. Corticosteroids alone or in combination with cyclosporine or cyclophosphamide are first-line therapies.

QUESTION 4

✴ What is the characteristic clinical finding in chronic renal disease patients on hemodialysis who develop antierythropoietin antibodies?

A. Concurrent fall in platelets with worsening anemia
B. Increasing thrombocytosis with worsening anemia

C. Decrease in hemoglobin of 0.5 to 1.0 g/dL weekly or requirement of 1to 2 units of blood transfusion per week

D. Increasing lymphocytosis with worsening anemia

Answer: C. Decrease in Hgb of 0.5 to 1.0 g/dL weekly or requirement of 1 to 2 units of blood transfusion per week, along with normal platelets (platelet count may decrease but is usually in the normal range) and normal white blood cell count, is characteristic of anti-EPO antibody-related anemia. A rise in serum ferritin due to the decreased utilization of iron is also seen (*Eur J Haematol.* 2004;73(6):389).

CASE 72

A 22-year-old male patient presents with recurrent epistaxis and a history of prolonged bleeding after minor cuts. At age 4, he had a splenectomy due to presumed immune thrombocytopenia. He is referred to hematology for evaluation of thrombocytopenia. His platelet count is 47,000/μL. Hemoglobin and leukocyte counts are normal. A peripheral blood smear is shown below.

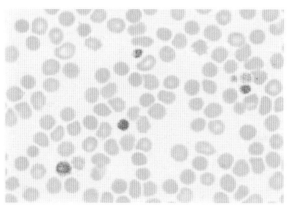

CASE FIGURE 72-1

QUESTION 1

☆ The clinical history and peripheral smear are consistent with a diagnosis of?

A. May–Hegglin anomaly
B. Wiskott–Aldrich syndrome
C. Glanzmann thrombasthenia
D. Platelet satellitisim
E. Bernard–Soulier syndrome (BSS)

Answer: E. The peripheral blood smear shows large/giant platelets. This finding, with the history of bleeding, is most consistent with a diagnosis of BSS. BSS is an inherited, usually autosomal recessive, platelet disorder characterized by prolonged bleeding time, thrombocytopenia, and large platelets. Of note, Howell–Jolly bodies and a few acanthocytes are also evident on the blood smear secondary to splenectomy. Immune thrombocytopenia (ITP) may resemble BSS in that platelets may be large.

However, the diagnosis of BSS can be established by flow cytometry, which revealed decreased surface GP1b and confirmed the diagnosis of BSS in our patient. Several patients with BSS have undergone splenectomy because of a misdiagnosis of ITP. Patients with May–Hegglin anomaly are usually asymptomatic and have no serious bleeding issues. Also, peripheral blood in these patients shows blue inclusions in the leukocytes plus large platelets. Wiskott–Aldrich syndrome is associated with small platelets, while platelets in Glanzmann thrombasthenia are of normal size. Platelet satellitism is an in vitro phenomenon and is thought to be related to the chemical EDTA in blood-collection tubes.

QUESTION 2

✫ What is the underlying defect in Bernard–Soulier syndrome?

A. GATA1 mutation
B. 3p21/NBEAL2 mutation
C. GPIIb/IIIa defect
D. GP1b/IX/V defect
E. Thrombospondin deficiency

Answer: D. BSS is caused by the absence of the GP1b/IX/V receptor complex on the surface of platelets, which is a critical receptor complex in hemostasis and thrombosis. This complex is the receptor for von Willebrand factor (vWF), and such defects result in deficient binding of vWF to the platelet membrane causing defective platelet adhesion. GATA1 mutations have been described in patients with an x-linked disorder who have thrombocytopenia and red cell abnormalities. NBEAL2 mutation has been noted in patients with the gray platelet syndrome. GPIIb/IIIa is a receptor target used in the treatment of coronary artery disease.

QUESTION 3

✫ What test can be used as a confirmatory laboratory finding in the evaluation of Bernard–Soulier syndrome?

A. Deficient ristocetin-dependent platelet agglutination
B. Deficient primary and secondary response to ADP
C. Normal agglutination studies
D. Deficient collagen-dependent platelet agglutination

Answer: A., Patients with BSS fail to aggregate with ristocetin and thus deficient ristocetin-dependent platelet aggregation is an indirect way to assess GPIb-IX-V/VWF interaction, which is the underlying defect in Bernard–Soulier syndrome (*Haematologica.* 2011;96:355–359).

QUESTION 4

✫ What treatment has limited effectiveness in the management of Bernard–Soulier syndrome?

A. Platelet transfusion
B. Antifibrinolytic agents
C. DDAVP (desmopressin)
D. Bone marrow transplantation

Answer: C. DDAVP is more useful in the treatment of platelet *function* defects than it is in conditions involving platelet receptor deficiency. This does not preclude a trial of desmopressin in BSS patients. Platelet transfusions are an integral part of the acute management of bleeding episodes but alloimmunization is a serious complication. Antifibrinolytics are useful for minor bleeding and prevention of postprocedure bleeding. Bone marrow transplantation has been successful in several patients with Bernard–Soulier syndrome. Recombinant factor VII has also been of benefit (*Br J Haematol.* 2010;149:813–823).

QUESTION 5

✫ What clinical finding is a contraindication to the use of antifibrinolytic agents?

A. History of ischemic stroke
B. Concurrent use of beta blockers
C. Hepatic dysfunction
D. Hematuria
E. Platelet refractoriness

Answer: D. Owing to the risk of clots causing genitourinary tract obstruction, the use of antifibrinolytic agents in patients with hematuria is not recommended.

CASE 73

A 34-year-old male patient is seen in hematology clinic to establish care. He states he has sickle cell disease. Complete blood count shows leukocyte count of 5,300/μL, hemoglobin 12.3 g/dL, MCV 77 fL, and platelet count 212,000/μL. The peripheral smear is shown below.

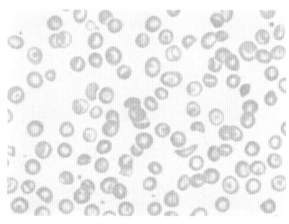

CASE FIGURE 73-1

QUESTION 1

✯ Hemoglobin electrophoresis is performed and shows equal portions of HbS and HbC, consistent with HbSC disease. Which of the following statements describes HbSC disease?

A. HbSC patients rarely have functional asplenia
B. HbSC patients experience the same spectrum of complications as HbSS patients, but at a decreased frequency
C. HbSC patients have a similar life expectancy to HbSS patients
D. Patients with HbSC disease have more treatment options than HbSS patients

Answer: B. Functional asplenia commonly occurs in HbSC patients, but at an advanced age compared with HbSS patients. HbSC patients have a lower incidence of the complications associated with HbSS disease. Life expectancy with SC is roughly 20 years longer than with SS. There are no treatment options for patients with SC that are unavailable to patients with SS disease (*J Clin Epidemiol.* 1992;45(8):893, *N Engl J Med.* 1994;330(23):1639).

QUESTION 2

✸ What red blood cell abnormality would not be expected on the peripheral smear in a patient with HbSC disease?

A. Howell–Jolly bodies
B. Target cells
C. Folded forms ("pita bread" or "clam-shell")
D. Sickle cells
E. Acanthocytes

Answer: E. Acanthocytes are not usually seen in patients with SC disease. As shown in the peripheral blood smear, many codocytes and a few sickle cells are seen. No acanthocytes are present. Howell–Jolly bodies may be present, especially in asplenic or hyposplenic SC patients. Target cells, folded forms, and sickle cells are all red cell findings evident in varying degrees in patients with HbSC disease (*Blood.* 1991;78(8):2104).

A 50-year-old man is admitted to the hospital with a fever, sore throat, and malaise. He has a past medical history of tobacco and substance abuse, including cocaine. Physical exam shows severe mouth ulcers, but is otherwise unremarkable with no organomegaly or lymphadenopathy. Laboratory studies reveal leukocyte count 1,200/μL, hemoglobin 14.6 g/dL, and platelet count 253,000/μL. The peripheral blood smear and bone marrow aspirate are shown below.

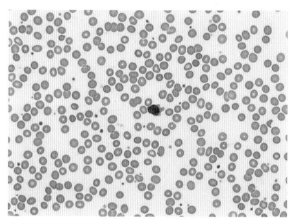

CASE FIGURE 74-1

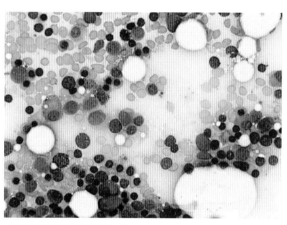

CASE FIGURE 74-2

QUESTION 1

☆ The peripheral blood smear reveals agranulocytosis, and the bone marrow aspirate shows a paucity of myeloid precursors with a maturation block at the promyelocyte stage, findings consistent with drug-induced agranulocytosis. Agranulocytosis is attributed to cocaine abuse. What is the proposed pathogenesis of this finding?

A. Direct marrow toxicity
B. Cocaine-associated autoantibodies
C. Hemolysis
D. Toxicity of agents mixed with cocaine

Answer: D. The drug levamisole, an immunomodulatory agent as well as an antihelminthic agent used in veterinary medicine, has been reported to be the putative cause agent of cocaine-induced agranulocytosis. Up to 69% of seized cocaine shipments have been found to contain this drug (*MMWR.* 2009;58(49):1381).

CASE 75

A 41-year-old African American female patient is referred for evaluation of leukopenia. She reports she is generally in good health, but she has noted increasing shortness of breath in recent weeks. She has a history of ovarian carcinoid tumor that was treated surgically. Complete blood count shows leukocyte count 2,100/μL, hemoglobin 12.2 g/dL, and platelet count 230,000/μL. Physical exam shows no splenomegaly or lymphadenopathy. Images below are from CT chest and bone marrow biopsy.

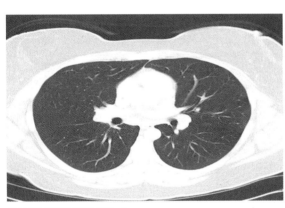

CASE FIGURE 75-1

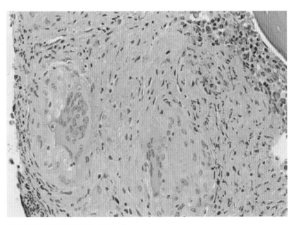

CASE FIGURE 75-2

QUESTION 1

☆ What is the most likely diagnosis?

A. Ovarian carcinoid metastatic to lung and bone
B. Sarcoidosis
C. Hodgkin lymphoma
D. Non-Hodgkin lymphoma

Answer: B. Sarcoidosis, especially when presenting with cytopenias and extrapulmonary involvement, can be found in the bone marrow as evidenced by the image above showing noncaseating granulomas. In addition, CT scan depicts bilateral hilar adenopathy. The other choices could be considered in the initial differential diagnosis of this patient, but are less consistent with the overall clinical presentation and bone marrow biopsy specimen.

QUESTION 2

✯ As part of the evaluation, serum angiotensin-converting enzyme (ACE) level is drawn. What statement is true regarding the use of ACE levels in sarcoidosis?

A. ACE levels are elevated in > 90% of patients with active sarcoidosis
B. ACE levels greater than 150% of normal correlate with extrapulmonary sarcoidosis
C. False positive results limit the usefulness of the assay in diagnosis and therapy
D. Patients taking amiodarone should hold the medication for 48 hours prior to testing

Answer: C. While false-positive ACE elevations are not frequently encountered, the frequency is great enough to argue against the usage of ACE level to guide firm decisions in the diagnosis or treatment of sarcoidosis. In general, the ACE level is elevated in around 75% of patients with active disease. No clear relationship between specific cutoffs in ACE elevation and extrapulmonary sarcoid has been demonstrated. Amiodarone does not affect the ACE level (*Ann Clin Biochem.* 1989;26(Pt 1):13).

CASE 76

A 32-year-old female patient is seen in the hematology clinic for follow-up of presumed ITP diagnosed during pregnancy 18 months previously. Complete blood count shows leukocyte count 7,000/μL, hemoglobin 13.8 g/dL, and platelet count 40,000/μL. She had been treated with prednisone, but did not respond. The peripheral blood smear is shown below.

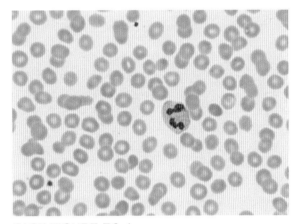

CASE FIGURE 76-1

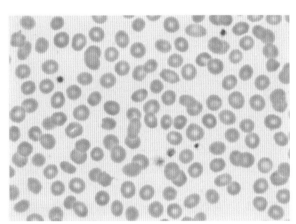

CASE FIGURE 76-2

QUESTION 1

⭐ Further family history is taken; the patient's mother, son, and brother all have platelet counts in the 70,000/μL to 90,000/μL range. Which of the following is the most likely diagnosis?

A. Gestational thrombocytopenia
B. Fanconi anemia
C. Immune thrombocytopenia
D. May–Hegglin anomaly

Answer: D. The peripheral blood smear shows large platelets and a leukocyte with a blue inclusion, which is characteristic of May–Hegglin anomaly. May–Hegglin anomaly is one of the four "MYH9-related macrothrombocytopenia disorders," the other three syndromes being Fechtner, Sebastian, and Epstein. MYH9-related disease is one of the most common types of inherited thrombocytopenia. It is an autosomal dominant disorder due to mutations of MYH9, the gene for the heavy chain of nonmuscle myosin IIA. Thrombocytopenia is usually mild and may be due to defects in

168

megakaryocyte maturation and platelet formation. The diagnosis should be suspected when giant platelets are seen on the blood smear and can be confirmed by an immunofluorescence test on the blood film.

QUESTION 2

★ What extrahematologic disorders may affect patients with MYH9-related diseases?

A. Renal dysfunction, cataracts, hearing impairment
B. Atypical infections, increased risk of lymphoma, eczema
C. Hearing impairment, cardiac defects, increased risk of lymphoma
D. Developmental delay, hearing impairment, cardiac defects

Answer: A. Renal dysfunction, cataracts, and deafness are associated with the MYH9-related diseases, and affect 30%, 16%, and 60% of patients, respectively. Genotype/phenotype correlations have been recognized, and therefore mutation screening is beneficial to help define the risk of acquiring such conditions (*Br J Haematol*. 2011;154:161–174).

CASE 77

A 76-year-old female patient is referred to hematology clinic for evaluation of persistent monocytosis. CBC reveals leukocyte count of 9,600/μL with absolute monocyte count 1200/μL, hemoglobin 11.3 g/dL, MCV 88 fL, and platelet count 257,000/μL. Physical exam is normal. The peripheral blood smear is shown below.

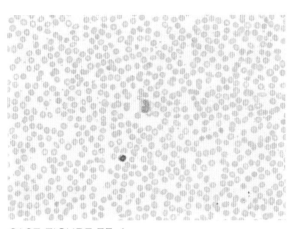

CASE FIGURE 77-1

QUESTION 1

☆ What disorder is not typically associated with monocytosis?

A. Folate deficiency
B. Sarcoidosis
C. Infections
D. Lymphoma
E. Chronic liver disease

Answer: A. Folate deficiency is associated with macrocytic red cells and hypersegmented neutrophils. The remaining disorders represent a partial list of conditions that may be associated with monocytosis.

QUESTION 2

✵ After viewing the peripheral blood smear and finding Howell–Jolly bodies, codocytes, and acanthocytes, further history is elicited from the patient that she had splenectomy after a car accident 30 years previously. What red blood cell abnormality is not usually noted in the red cells of a patient post splenectomy?

A. Howell–Jolly bodies
B. Target cells
C. Acanthocytes
D. Pappenheimer bodies
E. Echinocytes

Answer: E. All of the above choices except echinocytes may be seen in the peripheral blood of patients after splenectomy. Echinocytes (also called burr cells) can represent artifacts or may be associated with end-stage renal disease.

QUESTION 3

✵ What finding involving the white blood cell counts is common post splenectomy?

A. Decreased eosinophils
B. Decreased neutrophils
C. Increased lymphocytes
D. Decreased lymphocytes

Answer: C. The lymphocyte count is commonly increased following splenectomy, and some patients have even been suspected of harboring a lymphoproliferative disorder, such as lymphocytic leukemia (CLL), after splenectomy. However, flow cytometry of the lymphocytes post splenectomy are polyclonal, whereas in CLL, they are monoclonal.

A 78-year-old female patient presents with fatigue and weakness. On physical exam, she has splenomegaly. CBC shows leukocyte count of 15,400/μL with 38% monocytes and 22% eosinophils; hemoglobin is 10.3 g/dL and platelet count is 143,000/μL. The blood smear is depicted below.

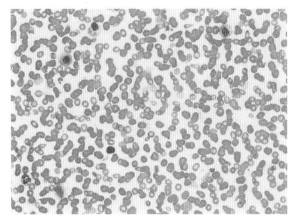

CASE FIGURE 78-1

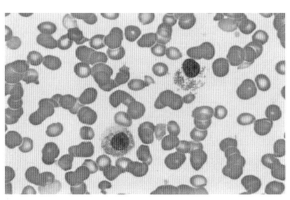

CASE FIGURE 78-2

QUESTION 1

✫ Based on the clinical presentation and above laboratory results, a diagnosis of chronic myelo-monocytic leukemia (CMML) is considered. Which of the following tests is most important in the diagnostic evaluation of this disease?

A. Evaluation for BCR-ABL fusion gene
B. FISH for trisomy 8
C. FISH for isochromosome 17q
D. JAK2 mutation

Answer: A. The peripheral blood smear shows monocytosis and increased eosinophils, and a few eosinophils demonstrate hyposegmented nuclei and hypogranulation. Basophilia and a myeloid left shift are not evident. Nonetheless, a positive test for the presence of the Philadelphia chromosome gene fusion product BCR-ABL would be consistent with chronic myeloid leukemia, rather than CMML, and thus a negative finding for this gene is part of the diagnostic criteria of CMML. In addition, a positive test would diagnose chronic myelogenous leukemia, and the treatment would be different from that of CMML. Trisomy 8 and isochromosome 17q are genetic aberrations associated with a hematologic disorder referred to as "atypical CML." JAK2 mutation is positive in patients with myeloproliferative neoplasms, but only in a small minority of patients with CMML.

QUESTION 2

⭑ Further testing reveals a t(5;12)(q33-q13;p12) translocation. What gene rearrangement is associated with this translocation?

A. RUNX1
B. NOTCH1
C. HOX11
D. PDGFRB

Answer: D. t(5;12)(q31-q33;p12) is associated with the formation of an PDGRB-ETV6 fusion gene, which has been reported in association with CMML, usually with eosinophilia. The WHO classification includes a category for rearrangements affecting PDGFRA, PDGFRB, or FGFR1. This is a separate entity from CMML, which is now included in the category of "myeloproliferative/myelodysplastic neoplasms." RUNX1 is associated with AML, whereas NOTCH1 and HOX11 have been found to play a role in T-lymphoblastic leukemia/lymphoma.

QUESTION 3

⭑ Testing for PDGFRB returns positive. What is the most appropriate treatment for this patient?

A. Azacitidine
B. Daunorubicin with cytarabine
C. Etoposide
D. Imatinib
E. Sunitinib

Answer: D. Patients with CMML harboring PDGFRB translocations exhibit durable responses with the use of imatinib, which is considered the most appropriate therapy in the nonemergent setting in cases harboring PDGFRB translocations (*NEJM*. 2002;347(7):481, *Blood*. 2002;100(3):1088, *Blood*. 2007;109(1):61).

CASE 79

A 32-year-old female patient presents with fatigue and dyspnea. She appears pale, but has an otherwise normal physical examination. Complete blood count shows leukocyte count 195,000/μL, hemoglobin 6.8 g/dL, and platelet count 10,000/μL. The peripheral blood smear is shown below.

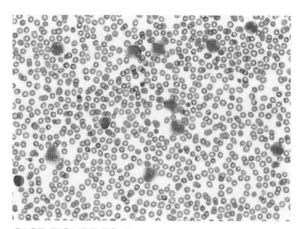

CASE FIGURE 79-1

QUESTION 1

✵ What findings on the peripheral blood smear would be consistent with a diagnosis of acute myeloid leukemia?

A. Absent nucleoli, coarse chromatin, stains positive for peroxidase
B. Prominent nucleoli, coarse chromatin, stains positive for peroxidase
C. Absent nucleoli, fine chromatin, negative peroxidase staining
D. Prominent nucleoli, fine chromatin, stains positive for peroxidase

Answer: D. AML blasts have prominent nucleoli and fine chromatin and may stain positive for peroxidase.

QUESTION 2

✷ Based on the following peripheral blood smear and bone marrow images, what is the most likely diagnosis?

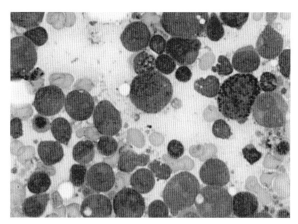

CASE FIGURE 79-2

A. Acute myeloid leukemia with t(8:21)
B. Acute myeloid leukemia monosomy −5 or −7
C. Acute myeloid leukemia with inv(16)
D. Acute myeloid leukemia with t(9;11)

Answer: C. The blood smear shows immature appearing monocytes as well as myeloid blasts. The bone marrow aspirate shows eosinophilic myeloid precursors with coarse basophilic granules. Such findings are characteristic of AML with inv(16). FISH for inv(16) was positive and confirmed a diagnosis of AML inv(16). The inv(16) is a pericentric inversion of chromosome 16, involving core binding factor and muscle myosin heavy chain genes. AML with inv(16) is recognized as a distinct clinical entity with a favorable prognosis and accounts for 6% to 8% of all cases of AML. As shown in the blood smear, there is usually leukocytes with monocytic and granulocytic differentiation. In addition, the bone marrow shows a variable number of immature eosinophils with striking granules. AML with t(8;21) also has a favorable prognosis, but has a different morphologic appearance, which, in many cases, includes the presence of needle-like Auer rods. AML with monosomy −5 or −7 and AML with t(9;11) are therapy-related and carry a relatively poor prognosis (*NEJM*. 1983;309:630–636).

QUESTION 3

✷ What clinical scenario is associated with AML with inv(16)?

A. Young patient with extramedullary myeloid sarcoma
B. Elderly patient with massive splenomegaly
C. Young patient with abdominal lymphadenopathy
D. Elderly patient with renal failure due to tumor lysis syndrome

Answer: A. AML with inv(16) may be associated with extramedullary involvement and indeed has been reported in 10% to 20% of patients. Chemotherapy and radiation may be used in the management of extramedullary AML. The prognostic significance of extramedullary AML is not well defined (*JCO.* 1995; 13(7):1800–1816, *Blood.* 2011;118(14):3785–3793).

QUESTION 4

✫   What is the standard approach for treatment in favorable-risk acute myeloid leukemia in a young, healthy patient?

A. Immediate referral for bone marrow transplantation
B. Observation in the case of extramedullary-only disease until symptoms occur
C. Standard induction therapy with cytarabine and an anthracycline
D. Single-agent azacitidine

Answer: C. Favorable risk AML is treated with cytarabine and an anthracycline (7 + 3). Bone marrow transplantation is used in relapsed or refractory AML, in patients obtaining second remission, or in some patients with intermediate-risk AML in first remission. Extramedullary AML should be treated rather than observed. Azacitidine is sometimes used as a single agent in the treatment of elderly patients with AML.

CASE 80

A 50-year-old female patient presents for evaluation of pancytopenia. She has hepatitis C. Laboratory evaluation shows leukocyte count 3,100/μL, hemoglobin 10.8 g/dL, and platelet count 78,000/μL. Physical exam is notable for splenomegaly. The peripheral smear is shown below.

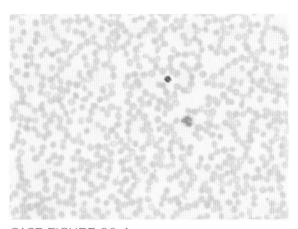

CASE FIGURE 80-1

QUESTION 1

★ What is the typical peripheral blood smear findings in a patient with hypersplenism?

A. Howell–Jolly bodies and hyposegmented neutrophils
B. Normal blood cells
C. Giant platelets
D. Nucleated red cells
E. Tear drop red cells

Answer: B. As depicted in the above image, the blood smear is usually normal in most patients with hypersplenism, although comorbid disease may cause the appearance of abnormal forms. Howell–Jolly bodies are seen in splenectomized patients and in cases of hemolytic anemia or megaloblastic anemia. Hyposegmented neutrophils are seen in myelodysplastic syndromes (MDS). Giant platelets indicate a marrow response to peripheral destruction of cells or may be seen in MDS and myeloproliferative neoplasms. Nucleated RBCs may be observed in myelophthisic conditions, as well as acute hemolytic anemia, acute hemorrhage, and several other hematologic disorders. Tear drop red blood cells (dacrocytes) are seen with myelophthisic anemia and with extramedullary hematopoiesis.

CASE 81

A 43-year-old female patient is referred for evaluation of leukocytosis which has been present for the last 3 years. Complete blood shows leukocyte count of 17,000, hemoglobin 14.3 g/dL, and platelet count 390,000/μL. Physical exam shows no lymphadenopathy or hepatosplenomegaly. Other than a long history of tobacco abuse, the patient has no significant medical problems. The peripheral blood smear is shown below.

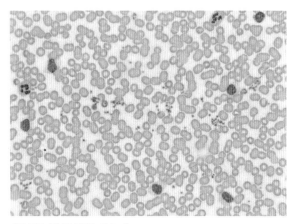

CASE FIGURE 81-1

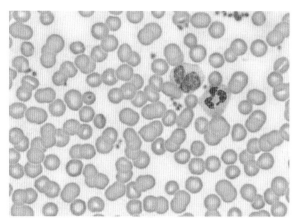

CASE FIGURE 81-2

QUESTION 1

⭐ Which of the following tests would be the next appropriate step in the evaluation of this patient?

A. Flow cytometry
B. Bone marrow biopsy
C. Stain for myeloperoxidase
D. Stain for nonspecific esterase
E. TCR gene rearrangement

Answer: A. The peripheral blood smear shows large lymphocytes with clumped chromatin, some of which have bilobed nuclei, without azurophilic cytoplasmic granules. This finding, coupled with a smoking history in a female, should make one consider polyclonal lymphocytois, which has been described in such patients. Flow cytometry would be critical to determine if the expansion in white cells is monoclonal or polyclonal. Bone marrow biopsy might be indicated depending on the results of flow cytometry. Myeloperoxidase and nonspecific esterase staining may be used in the diagnosis of acute myeloid leukemia (AML) but has been supplanted by flow cytometry. TCR gene rearrangement assay is of value in the evaluation of large granular lymphocytes (LGL) leukemia, which is usually associated with neutropenia and large lymphocytes with prominent granules.

QUESTION 2

✭   What flow cytometry results would be consistent with a polyclonal B-cell population?

A. Positivity for CD3 and FMC7
B. Positivity for CD19 and FMC7, both kappa and lambda light chains expressed
C. Positivity for CD3 and CD19, both kappa and lambda light chains expressed
D. Positivity for CD5 and CD19, no expression of kappa or lambda light chains

Answer: B. Both CD19 and FMC7 are B-cell markers. CD3 is a T-cell marker, and CD5 may be found on both B and T cells. In a polyclonal lymphocyte population, both kappa and lambda light chains would be expressed.

QUESTION 3

✭   The patient is diagnosed with persistent polyclonal B-cell lymphocytosis (PPBL). Which of the following is true regarding this condition?

A. Binucleated lymphocytes are a rare finding; smoking cessation leads to resolution of the lymphocytosis
B. Binucleated lymphocytes are a common finding; smoking cessation does not lead to resolution of the lymphocytosis
C. Binucleated lymphocytes are a common finding; smoking cessation leads to resolution of the lymphocytosis
D. Binucleated lymphocytes are a rare finding; smoking cessation does not lead to resolution of the lymphocytosis

Answer: B. Binucleated lymphocytes are a common finding (making up 1.5% to 9% of lymphocytes). Smoking cessation does not lead to resolution of the lymphocytosis (*Br J Haematol.* 1999; 104: 486–493).

CASE 82

An 81-year-old male patient presents with a 4-month history of progressive purple skin lesions on his face, trunk, and lower extremities. Complete blood count shows leukocyte count 4,400/μL, hemoglobin 10.6 g/dL, and platelet count 188,000/μL. LDH was elevated at 482 U/L. The peripheral blood smear is shown below.

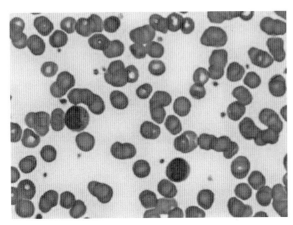

CASE FIGURE 82-1   CASE FIGURE 82-2

QUESTION 1

☆ Flow cytometry of the peripheral blood shows expression of CD2, CD8, CD43, and CD56 and lack of expression for CD3, CD4, CD16, and CD57. These results are most consistent with what type of cell population?

A. Plasma cells
B. Natural killer (NK) cells
C. Myeloid blasts
D. Lymphoid blasts

Answer: B. CD2+, surface CD3−, and CD56+ is consistent with an NK-cell population. The peripheral blood shows medium and large cells with basophilic cytoplasm, and fine chromation and a nucleolus in the large cell; azurophilic granules can be observed in the cytoplasm. The patient developed progressive skin lesions with a rapid increase in leukocytes, with large immature cells and worsening thrombocytopenia and anemia. A diagnosis of aggressive natural killer cell leukemia was established.

CASE 83

A 9-month-old male patient is referred by his pediatrician due to an abnormal blood count. Leukocyte count is 7,300/µL, hemoglobin is 7.4 g/dL with MCV 109 fL, reticulocytes is 1.0%, and platelet count is 581,000/µL. The physical examination reveals no abnormal findings. The peripheral blood smear shows mild macrocytosis but is otherwise unremarkable. The image below shows the bone marrow aspirate specimen.

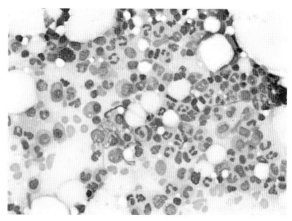

CASE FIGURE 83-1

QUESTION 1

✫ Diamond–Blackfan anemia or transient erythroblastopenia of childhood (TEC) are considered in the differential diagnosis. Which of the following choices is correct in describing the findings that would support a diagnosis of Diamond–Blackfan anemia (DBA)?

A. DBA is more likely to be diagnosed after 1 year of age, whereas TEC is diagnosed before age 1 in most cases
B. TEC is more likely to be macrocytic
C. HbF is usually increased in patients with DBA
D. Erythrocyte adenosine demaminase (ADA) levels are elevated in TEC

Answer: C. The image shows a normocellular marrow with decreased to absent red cell precursors. This could represent either DBA or TEC. Several factors can be used to differentiate these two disorders including the following: DBA usually occurs before age 1, the anemia is macrocytic, HbF is elevated, and erythrocyte ADA is elevated (*Br J Haematol.* 2008;142:859–876).

QUESTION 2

☆ What condition is not a congenital abnormality associated with patients who have Diamond–Blackfan anemia?

A. Microcephaly
B. Papillomatous skin lesions
C. Syndactyly
D. Absent or horseshoe kidney
E. Short neck

Answer: B. The list of congenital abnormalities associated with DBA is extensive but does not include papillomatous skin lesions. Craniofacial abnormalities predominate. Not all patients with DBA have apparent abnormalities; the range in published studies of patients with DBA who have at least one definite abnormality is 35% to 47% (*Br J Haematol.* 2008;142:859–876).

QUESTION 3

☆ What is the pathophysiologic defect in DBA?

A. Defective telomerase enzyme
B. Defective ribosome synthesis
C. Mutation in colony stimulating factor gene
D. Sensitivity to apoptosis due to defective surface receptor proteins

Answer: B. DBA is caused by failure of hematopoiesis due to ineffective ribosomal proteins. Multiple genes have been implicated in DBA, including RPS19 in 25% of patients. In one study of 219 patients, 129 distinct mutations were found. Haploinsufficiency for ribosomal protein genes may cause activation of *p53* in erythroid progenitor cells in DBA (*ISO Hum Mutat.* 2010;31(12):1269). (*Blood.* 2011;117:2567–2576).

QUESTION 4

☆ What statement is true regarding the prognosis and treatment of Diamond–Blackfan anemia?

A. Survival at age 40 is less than 30%
B. Chemotherapy is considered second-line treatment
C. Matched sibling stem cell transplant results have been disappointing
D. Spontaneous remissions occur in 20% of patients
E. Corticosteroids should only be used intermittently

Answer: D. About 20% of patients have been reported to have spontaneous remission of DBA. The remissions are most likely to occur before age 10, and most remissions are durable. Chemotherapy does not have a role in the treatment of DBA. Matched sibling stem cell transplant is often successful and is considered a first-line therapy. Corticosteroids have been a mainstay in the treatment of DBA for decades and are often used for a prolonged period, which makes monitoring for side effects a major aspect of therapy (*Br J Haematol.* 2008;142:859–876).

A 21-year-old man is seen in the hematology clinic for evaluation of pancytopenia. The onset was noted at age 12, and the course has been progressive. Current leukocyte count is 2,100/μL, hemoglobin 8.4 g/dL with MCV 98 fL, and platelet count 29,000/μL. Reticulocyte percentage is decreased at 1.2% of red blood cells. On physical exam, he is noted to have short stature and multiple café-au-lait spots. While shaking his hand, you note that he has no thumb. The peripheral blood smear and bone marrow biopsy are shown below.

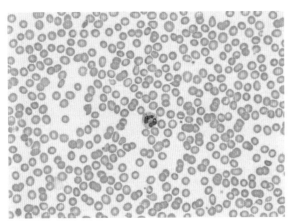

CASE FIGURE 84-1

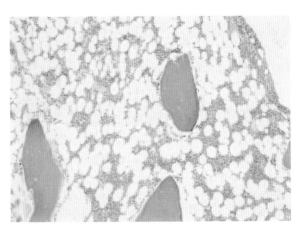

CASE FIGURE 84-2

QUESTION 1

★ What is the most likely diagnosis?

A. Dyskeratosis congenita
B. Shwachman–Diamond syndrome
C. Fanconi anemia
D. Amegakaryocytic thrombocytopenia

Answer: C. The blood smear reveals pancytopenia with mild macrocytosis, dacrocytes, and thrombocytopenia, and the bone marrow biopsy is hypocellular for the patient's age. Fanconi anemia (FA) is an autosomal and x-linked recessive disorder characterized by bone marrow failure, acute myelogenous leukemia, solid malignant neoplasms, and developmental abnormalities. FA should be considered in patients with pancytopenia and congenital anomalies. Radial bone and thumb abnormalities, short stature, and skin abnormalities are the most common manifestation of FA. Dyskeratosis congenita is associated with nail dystrophy, oral leukoplakia, and skin hyperpigmentation. Scwachman–Diamond syndrome is associated with exocrine pancreatic dysfunction and skeletal abnormalities. Amegakaryocytic thrombocytopenia does not have associated developmental or organ dysfunction.

QUESTION 2

✮ What is the underlying pathophysiologic mechanism of FA?

A. Defective mismatch repair genes
B. Abnormal chromosomal breakage
C. Dysregulation of telomerase
D. Faulty mitotic spindle formation

Answer: B. The primary molecular defect underlying FA is that cells derived from FA patients display hypersensitivity to DNA cross-linking agents, such as mitomycin-C and diepoxybutane, causing chromosomal breakage. The FA pathway is composed of at least 15 genes, and multiple genes have been identified as defective in patients with FA, the most common being FA-A, located on chromosome 16. Mismatch repair defects are seen in some types of colorectal cancer. Telomerase function is defective in dyskeratosis congenita. Mitotic spindle stabilization may play a role in the pathophysiologic mechanism of Scwachman–Diamond syndrome, but this is not well understood.

QUESTION 3

✮ What type of malignancy is NOT commonly associated with FA?

A. Myelodysplastic syndrome (MDS)
B. Acute lymphocytic leukemia (ALL)
C. Acute myeloid leukemia (AML)
D. Squamous cell cancer of the head and neck (SCCHN)

Answer: B. AML, MDS, and SCCHN are all associated with FA; the incidence of hematologic malignancy is 33% and the incidence of nonhematologic malignancy is 28% by age 40. The cases of AML are usually M1-M4 FAB subtype and do not have any characteristic molecular abnormality. Of note, patients with AML cannot be treated with standard doses of alkylating agents; they have marked increased toxicity with such agents. Likewise, stem cell transplantation in these patients is associated with many challenges. Bone marrow failure is a common cause of death and occurs in up to 90% of FA patients by age 40 (*Hem Onc Cl N Am*. 2009;23:193–214).

QUESTION 4

⭐ What treatment approach is warranted in patients with FA?

A. Observation, followed by androgen administration with the onset of moderate bone marrow failure
B. Bone marrow transplantation (BMT) at the time of diagnosis if there is an appropriate donor available
C. Observation, followed by the use of hematopoietic growth factors
D. Systemic chemotherapy at the time of diagnosis

Answer: A. Patients with mild bone marrow failure may be observed closely. With the onset of moderate bone marrow failure (ANC 500 to 1,000, platelets 30,000–50,000/μL, and hemoglobin < 8 g/dL), androgens are given if BMT is not desirable or if there is not an appropriate donor. Treatment with BMT at the time of diagnosis has not been shown to improve outcomes.

A 48-year-old woman is seen for evaluation of thrombocytopenia. She has no history of abnormal bleeding. She has a history of IV drug abuse. On physical exam, there is no lymphadenopathy or palpable splenomegaly. Complete blood count (CBC) shows leukocyte count of 6,700/μL, hemoglobin 13.7 g/dL, and platelet count 46,000/μL. The peripheral blood smear is shown below.

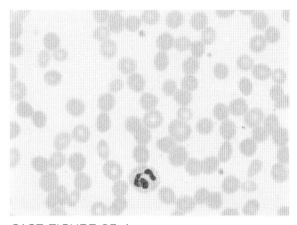

CASE FIGURE 85-1

QUESTION 1

☆ Due to the patient's history of IV drug use, a hepatitis panel and HIV tests are ordered. What would be an appropriate next step in the management of the patient?

A. Bone marrow biopsy
B. Flow cytometry of peripheral blood
C. Liver–spleen scan
D. Antiplatelet antibody assay

Answer: C. The blood smear shows decreased platelets but normal leukocytes and red cells. Nuclear medicine liver–spleen scan can determine the function of the liver and spleen and thus can assess for the presence of hypersplenism, which, if present, would indicate that platelet sequestration is at least a contributor to thrombocytopenia in this case.

QUESTION 2

✻ The liver–spleen scan does not show hypersplenism. Laboratory results reveal chronic hepatitis C infection. What is the most likely mechanism of thrombocytopenia in this case?

A. Decreased thrombopoietin production
B. Direct marrow suppression from the viral infection
C. Immune-mediated platelet destruction
D. Platelet sequestration despite normal spleen size

Answer: C. In this patient, who has normal liver function and no other cytopenias, immune-mediated platelet destruction secondary to hepatitis C infection is the most likely etiology. Platelet autoantibodies have been detected in 66% of HCV-infected individuals. Choices A and B represent causes of thrombocytopenia, which would be prominent in advanced cases of hepatitis C infection (*Br J Haematol.* 2005;129:818–824).

CASE 86

A 22-year-old female who immigrated from Gabon, Africa, 3 years ago presented to the hospital with sudden pain in her right eye. She also felt that something was moving in her sclera. She denied fever, chills, night sweats, weight loss, rash, or swelling. Laboratory evaluation showed a leukocyte count of 9,100/μL with 22% eosinophils, hemoglobin 13.0 g/dL, and platelet 328,000/μL. The peripheral blood smear is shown below.

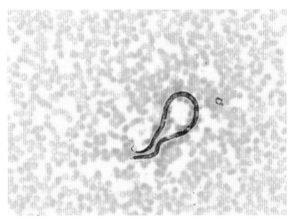

CASE FIGURE 86-1

QUESTION 1

☆ What is the most likely diagnosis?

A. Strongyloides
B. Onchorcerciasis
C. Mansonella infection
D. *Loa loa*

Answer: D. The peripheral blood smear shows an obvious microfilaria, and in light of the patient's ethnic background, is most likely *Loa loa*. Loiasis, known as the African eye worm, is caused by the filarial nematode *Loa loa* and is transmitted by the bite of the female Chrysops fly, which is endemic in the rain forest of Central and West Africa. After infection, the filarial nematode may migrate across the subconjunctiva of the eye and produce pain and swelling (Calabar swellings). Microfilariae may be detected in the blood smear and are usually 3 to 7 cm in length, as seen in the image. Of note, finger stick specimens may provide a better yield of microfilariae than do peripheral venipunctures, whereas late night blood draws are needed to detect nocturnal *Wuchereria bancrofti* and *Brugia malayi* (*Clin Lab Med.* 1991;11:977–1010).

QUESTION 2

✭ What coinfection would be important in the clinical management of this patient?

A. Strongyloides
B. Malaria
C. Onchocerciasis
D. Leishmaniasis

Answer: C. Coinfection with onchocerciasis should be considered, since treatment with diethylcarmazine may elicit serious inflammatory responses in the eye and skin. This patient was treated with albendazole.

A 19-year-old female patient of Greek heritage presents for evaluation of anemia. She is 7 months pregnant. Complete blood count (CBC) shows leukocyte count of 5,400/μL, hemoglobin 8.8 g/dL with MCV 62.7 fL, and platelet count 251,000/μL. The peripheral smear is shown below.

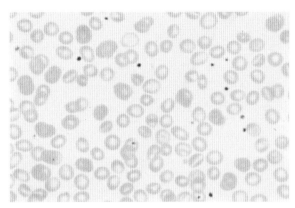

CASE FIGURE 87-1

QUESTION 1

★ What would support a diagnosis of beta thalassemia trait rather than simple iron deficiency?

A. Elevated RBC count
B. Elevated mean corpuscular hemoglobin concentration
C. Elevated red cell distribution width (RDW)
D. Decreased RBC count

Answer: A. A consistent finding in carriers of beta thalassemia is microcytic anemia with an elevated RBC count. The blood smear shows microcytic hypochromic red cells and target cells. Iron-deficiency anemia is associated with an increased RDW and decreased RBC counts (*Am J Public Health.* 1988 November;78(11):1476–1477).

QUESTION 2

☆ What finding on hemoglobin electrophoresis is consistent with beta thalassemia trait?

A. HbA-80%, HbA2 20%
B. HbA-80%, HbF-10%, HbA2-10%
C. HbA2-85%, HbF-15%
D. HbA-95%, HbA2-5%

Answer: D. HbA2 is increased in beta thalassemia trait, with values ranging from 3.5% to 7% (mean, 5%). HbF is increased in approximately 50% of patients, but the values observed are in the range of 1% to 3%.

A 53-year-old female patient is seen for evaluation prior to a planned dental extraction. She has systemic lupus erythematosus and has been noted to be thrombocytopenic on recent laboratory evaluation by her rheumatologist. The peripheral smear is shown below.

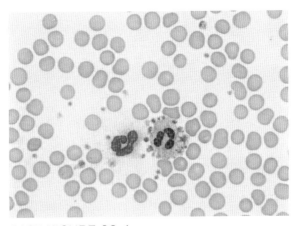

CASE FIGURE 88-1

QUESTION 1

★ What is the mechanism of this patient's thrombocytopenia?

A. Autoantibodies related to EDTA anticoagulant
B. Antiphospholipid antibodies
C. Antinuclear antibodies
D. Warm autoantibodies

Answer: A. The blood smear shows numerous platelets surrounding granulocytes, that is, platelet satellitism, a cause of pseudothrombocytopenia. This scenario is an in vitro phenomenon probably related to interactions between platelet glycoprotein IIb/IIIa complex and the neutrophil Fc receptor, caused by the anticoagulant EDTA contained in some blood collection containers. Platelet satellitism is less common than platelet clumping, also related to pseudothrombocytopenia (*N Engl J Med.* 1998;338:591).

CASE 89

A 54-year-old male patient is being evaluated for a lung mass seen on a CT scan for chest pain. He is otherwise healthy and his physical exam is normal. Complete blood count shows leukocyte count 5,700/μL, hemoglobin 14.2 g/dL, and platelet count 289,000/μL. The peripheral blood smear is shown below.

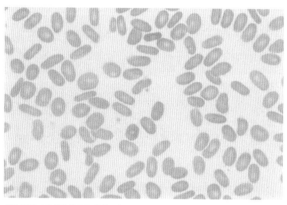

CASE FIGURE 89-1

QUESTION 1

☆ Based on the patient's history and peripheral blood smear, which of the following statements is most likely?

A. Hereditary elliptocytosis, which is most commonly inherited as an autosomal dominant condition
B. Hereditary spherocytosis, which is most commonly inherited as an autosomal recessive condition
C. Hereditary elliptocytosis, which is most commonly inherited as an autosomal recessive condition
D. Hereditary pyropoikilocytosis, which is most commonly inherited as an autosomal recessive condition

Answer: A. The blood smear shows that the majority of RBCs are biconcave elliptocytes consistent with a diagnosis of hereditary elliptocytosis (HE). HE is usually an autosomal dominant disorder and is most commonly asymptomatic. Elliptocytes may be found in iron deficiency, megaloblastic anemia, thalassemia, myelodysplasia, and myelofibrosis. However, in contrast to HE, the percentage of elliptocytes in these disorders does not usually exceed 40% to 50%.

QUESTION 2

✶ What is the pathophysiologic difference between hereditary spherocytosis (HS) and HE?

A. HE involves vertical protein interactions, most commonly affecting ankyrin
B. HE involves horizontal protein interactions, most commonly affecting spectrin
C. HS involves horizontal protein interactions, most commonly affecting spectrin
D. HS involves vertical protein interactions, most commonly affecting band 3

Answer: B. The principal defect in HE is a mechanical weakness or fragility of the erythrocyte membrane, primarily involving horizontal protein interactions, especially spectrin–spectrin and spectrin–protein 4.1 and the lipid bilayer. On the other hand, HS involves abnormalities of vertical protein interactions, especially ankyrin and ankyrin–spectrin.

A 38-year-old male patient is evaluated for fatigue. He has no other specific complaints; he denies fever, chills, abdominal pain, and urinary symptoms. Family history includes a brother who died at age of 8 years of renal failure. Complete blood count shows leukocyte count of 7,800/μL, hemoglobin 8.9 g/dL, and platelet count 9,000/μL. Creatinine is 7.9 mg/dL. LDH is 2200 U/L. The peripheral blood smear is shown below.

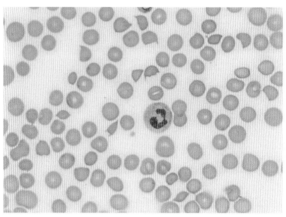

CASE FIGURE 90-1

QUESTION 1

★ This peripheral blood smear would be consistent with all of the following conditions except:

A. Thrombotic-thrombocytopenic purpura (TTP)
B. Malignant hypertension
C. Autoimmune hemolytic anemia (AIHA)
D. Disseminated intravascular coagulation (DIC)
E. Hemolytic uremic syndrome (HUS)

Answer: C. The peripheral smear is notable for the presence of schistocytes and thrombocytopenia. Schistocytes are characteristic of conditions associated with microangiopathic hemolytic anemia (MAHA). MAHA has been noted in patients with malignant hypertension, DIC, HUS, and several other disorders. However, MAHA is not usually observed in autoimmune hemolytic anemia, which is characterized by spherocytes in the peripheral blood smear. The clinical findings of MAHA, thrombocytopenia, renal failure, and a family history of renal failure in a sibling who died at a young age aroused suspicion for atypical HUS. Additional studies revealed a deficiency of complement factor H (CFH), the plasma regulator of the alternate pathway, in the patient. Approximately 10% of cases of the HUS are classified as atypical, and less than 20% of cases of atypical HUS are familial. Mutations in CFH have a reported frequency of 40% to 45% of patients with familial atypical HUS. Gene mutations involving the complement regulatory proteins result in excessive complement activation, endothelial cell damage, and local accumulation of platelet-fibrin thrombi.

QUESTION 2

✭   A diagnosis of atypical hemolytic-uremic syndrome would note what complement abnormalities?

A. Normal C4, decreased C3 levels
B. Decreased C4 and C3 levels
C. Normal C4 and C3 levels
D. Increased C4, normal C3 levels

Answer: A. In the atypical HUS syndrome, complement tests show decreased C3 and a normal C4. This is caused by activation of the alternative complement pathway, in which C3 is cleaved but C4 is not. (*NEJM*. 2009;361:1676–1687).

QUESTION 3

✭   Which statement is true regarding atypical HUS?

A. Atypical HUS accounts for 60% of HUS cases in children
B. Non-Shigella gastrointestinal illness prodrome is usually present
C. Prognosis is better for atypical HUS than classic HUS
D. Infection and genetic mutations are both causes of atypical HUS

Answer: D. Atypical HUS cases account for about 10% of HUS in children. Although infections can precede atypical HUS, the diarrheal prodrome characteristic of HUS is usually not present. Patients with familial atypical HUS have a poor prognosis, with end-stage renal disease or death in 50% to 80% of patients. Sporadic atypical HUS may be caused by a variety of conditions, including infections, cancer and antineoplastic agents, pregnancy, systemic lupus, organ transplantation, and medications such as cyclosporine and ticlopidine.

QUESTION 4

✩ What treatment option is not part of the standard management of atypical HUS?

A. Cyclosporine
B. Combined kidney–liver transplantation
C. Eculizumab
D. Plasma exchange

Answer: A. Cyclosporine is not recommended in the treatment of typical or atypical HUS. Combined kidney–liver transplant is recommended for a subset of patients with high-risk genetic mutations. Eculizumab is a monoclonal antibody to human C5 and has been approved for use in atypical HUS. Plasma exchange may be utilized in the acute treatment of atypical HUS.

A 19-year-old male patient who is in remission after receiving 4 cycles of BEP chemotherapy for primary mediastinal yolk sac germ cell tumor presents with fatigue 3 months after his last cycle. Laboratory evaluation shows leukocyte count of 43,500/μL, hemoglobin 7.6 g/dL, and platelet count 7,000/μL. The peripheral blood smear is shown below. Flow cytometry of the peripheral blood cells express CD13, CD33, CD41, and CD61.

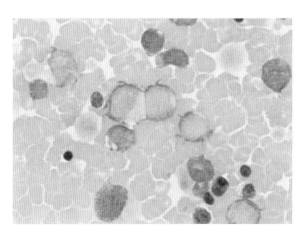

CASE FIGURE 91-1

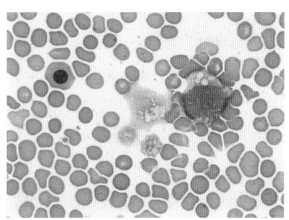

CASE FIGURE 91-2

QUESTION 1

☆ What is the most likely diagnosis?

A. Therapy-related acute lymphoblastic leukemia
B. Therapy-related acute myeloid leukemia
C. Acute megakaryoblastic leukemia
D. Therapy-related myelodysplastic syndrome evolving to acute leukemia

Answer: C. The blood smear shows large cells with fine chromatin, a high nuclear–cytoplasmic ratio, and cytoplasmic vacuoles and blebs; in addition, giant, hypogranular platelets are seen. Such blood findings in concert with the flow cytometry immunophenotype is characteristic of acute megakaryoblastic leukemia. Patients with primary nonseminomatous germ cell tumors, especially with a yolk sac component, have an increased incidence of hematologic malignancies, including acute leukemia and systemic mastocytosis, and acute megakaryoblastic leukemia is one of the most prevalent AML sub-types reported. The interval between the diagnosis of acute leukemia and germ cell tumor of 3 months contrasts with the average time of 24 to 60 months for therapy-related acute leukemia (*J Natl Cancer Inst.* 2000;92(1):54).

QUESTION 2

✺ What genetic aberration has been reported as a marker to determine the clonal relationship of primary mediastinal germ cell tumor and hematologic malignancies?

A. Deletion 11q23
B. Monosomy 7
C. Inv(16)
D. Isochromosome 12p

Answer: D. Although study numbers are small, multiple cases have reported isochromosome 12p in patients with hematologic malignancy and primary mediastinal nonseminaotous germ cell tumors. Isochromosome 12p has been detected in both the mediastinal tumor and underlying leukemia in the same patient, lending support to this hypothesis. This may be related to the fact that malignant germ cells have multipotential differentiation. Deletion 11q23 and monosomy 7 are aberrations seen in ther-apy-related disorders. Inv(16) is associated with favorable risk AML (*J Natl Cancer Inst.* 1990;82(3):221).

QUESTION 3

✺ What statement best describes the time interval and median survival of hematologic malignancies associated with primary mediastinal germ cell tumors?

A. Onset is usually 1 to 2 years and median survival 3 years
B. Onset is usually within 6 months and median survival is less than 6 months
C. Onset is usually 3 to 5 years and median survival less than 6 months
D. Onset is usually 1 to 2 years and median survival less than 6 months

Answer: B. The median time between the diagnosis of the tumor and the diagnosis of the hemato-logic malignancy is 5 months, and prognosis of these patients is extremely poor, with a median sur-vival of 1 month (range, 0 to 32) (*N Engl J Med.* 1990;322:1425–1429).

CASE 92

A 58-year-old man presents with generalized erythroderma with associated pruritis, weight loss, and cold intolerance. In addition to the generalized skin changes, he has generalized lymphadenopathy and hyperkeratosis of the palms and soles on physical exam. Complete blood count shows leukocyte count of 22,300/μL, hemoglobin 12.6 g/dL, and platelet count 164,000/μL. Peripheral blood smear is shown below.

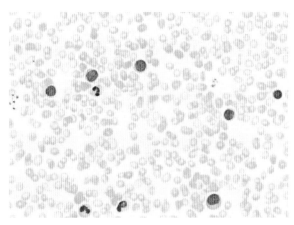

CASE FIGURE 92-1

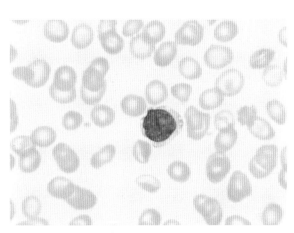

CASE FIGURE 92-2

QUESTION 1

★ What is the most likely diagnosis?

A. Sezary syndrome (SS)
B. Acute myeloid leukemia (AML)
C. Hairy cell leukemia (HCL)
D. Chronic lymphocytic leukemia (HCL)

Answer: A. The peripheral blood shows lymphocytes with condensed chromatin and "cerebriform" nuclei and vacuoles in the cytoplasm. This finding plus the patient's history and physical exam is characteristic of SS. Immunophenotype showed expression of CD2, CD3, and CD4 and lack of CD7. T-cell receptor (TCR) gene rearrangement was noted.

QUESTION 2

✭ Which finding is not included in making a diagnosis of SS?

A. Clonal TCR rearrangement in the peripheral blood
B. More than 1,000/μL Sezary cells in the peripheral blood
C. 80% skin involvement with erythroderma
D. CD8 positivity on immunophenotyping of a skin biopsy sample

Answer: D. Most patients with SS express CD4, although rare patients with SS are CD8+. The other three choices represent criteria used for the diagnosis of SS (*Blood.* 2007;110:1713).

QUESTION 3

✭ What is the most important clinical aspect affecting the prognosis of patients with SS?

A. Type of TCR gene rearrangement
B. Number of involved lymph node sites
C. Hyperkeratosis of palms and soles
D. Number of Sezary cells in the peripheral blood

Answer: D. The number of Sezary cells in the peripheral blood has been reported to be a significant prognostic factor (median OS of 7.6 years for patients with less than 1000/μL vs. 2.4 years for greater than 10,000/μL). Other factors that influence prognosis include advanced age, elevated LDH, and visceral involvement (*Int J Dermatol.* 2009;48(3):243–252).

A 39-year-old male patient is admitted to the ICU with chest pain, slurred speech, and left-sided weakness. Past medical history is significant for hypothyroidism, angina, and bipolar disorder. Home medications include valproic acid, levothyroxine, and sublingual nitroglycerin. On physical exam, he is in mild distress, afebrile, and mildly hypertensive. Complete blood count shows a leukocyte count of 6,600/μL, hemoglobin 6.5 g/dL, and platelet count 16,000/μL. Creatinine is 0.8 mg/dL and LDH is 683 U/L. Troponin level is normal. The peripheral blood smear is shown below.

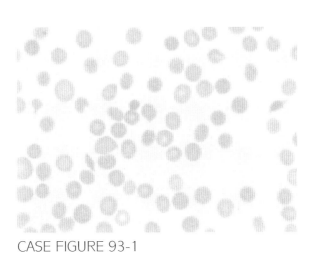

CASE FIGURE 93-1

QUESTION 1

★ What is the most important step in the management of this patient?

A. Begin high-dose steroids
B. Platelet transfusions to keep platelets > 30,000/μL
C. Plasma exchange
D. Neurology consultation

Answer: C. The peripheral blood smear shows schistocytes, helmet cells, polychromasia, and thrombocytopenia. Microangiopathic hemolytic anemia and thrombocytopenia should raise a suspicion for thrombotic thrombocytopenic purpura (TTP), and plasma exchange should be started immediately, due to the high mortality rate of untreated thrombotic thrombocytopenic purpura. Steroids have been included in the treatment of TTP, but are not as important as initiating plasma exchange. Platelet transfusions should be avoided unless there is significant bleeding, since it has been reported to be associated with an increased risk of thrombotic events. Neurology consultation would delay therapy unnecessarily.

QUESTION 2

✵ Which of the following statements is correct regarding ADAMTS13, the protease which has been found to play a pivotal role in TTP?

A. Low ADAMTS13 level predicts a poor response to plasma exchange
B. Low ADAMTS13 level identifies patients more likely to relapse early
C. Low ADAMTS13 level leads to an excess of small vWF multimers
D. Low ADAMTS13 level in acquired TTP is caused by Ig autoantibodies

Answer: B. Low levels of ADAMTS13 identify patients at high risk of early relapse; it is not predictive of a poor response to plasma exchange. ADAMTS13, a metalloprotease in plasma, cleaves vWF in plasma, and prevents vWF-mediated platelet aggregation. A deficiency of this protease leads to accumulation of ultra-large vWF multimers, which causes microvascular thrombosis in the heart, kidney, spleen, pancreas, adrenal gland, and brain. Such thrombi are composed of platelets and vWF, which is characteristic of TTP. IgG autoantibodies directed against ADAMTS13 are the primary pathogenetic mechanism involved in acquired TTP (*Blood.* 2010;115:1475–1476).

QUESTION 3

✵ The patient is treated with once daily plasma exchange and is started on methylprednisolone 125 mg TID. After 3 days, he is noted to have increasing confusion. LDH and platelet count are not improved. What would be an appropriate next plan of management?

A. Continue current management
B. Increase the frequency of plasma exchange to twice daily
C. Begin vincristine
D. Emergent splenectomy

Answer: B. Escalation of therapy is indicated when the patient shows clinical signs of deterioration. Increasing the frequency of plasma exchange has been shown to be effective. Chemotherapy and splenectomy are options for resistant cases, but these options are not commonly used as emergent options in the acute phase of management (*Transfusion.* 2007;48(2):349–357).

CASE 94

A 32-year-old female patient is seen in the hematology clinic for evaluation after her 6-year-old son was found to have abnormal blood cells. The pediatrician advised her to see a hematologist because her son may have a familial disorder. Neither the mother nor the son had any health problems. The patient's physical exam is normal. Laboratory studies show a leukocyte count of 9,600/μL, hemoglobin of 14.3 g/dL, and platelet count of 259,000/μL. The peripheral smear is shown below.

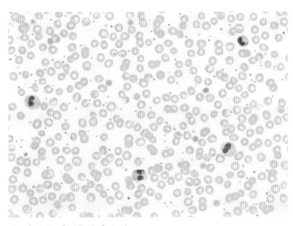

CASE FIGURE 94-1

QUESTION 1

★ What is the most likely diagnosis?

A. Shwachman–Diamond syndrome
B. Glanzmann thrombasthenia
C. Familial Pelger–Huet anomaly
D. Bernard–Soulier syndrome

Answer: C. The peripheral blood smear depicts neutrophils with bilobed, unilobed, or dumb-bell-shaped nuclei with dense chromatin, characteristic of the Pelger–Huet anomaly. Subsequent review of the son's blood smear revealed similar findings. Thus, a diagnosis of familial Pelger–Huet anomaly was established. Familial Pelger–Huet anomaly is a benign leukocyte anomaly that is inherited as an autosomal dominant trait. Patients with this disorder are asymptomatic, as the neutrophils have normal function. It is important to differentiate this familial condition from acquired Pelger–Huet anomaly associated with myelodysplastic syndromes (MDS). In the familial disorder, 80% to 90% of the neutrophils are abnormal, whereas in MDS only a minority of cells is usually evident. The other listed conditions are inherited conditions that primarily affect platelet function and are not associated with Pelger–Huet anomaly.

QUESTION 2

✫   What is the genetic aberration responsible for the Pelger–Huet anomaly?

A. Mutation in the lamin B receptor
B. Mutation in the concanavalin-A receptor
C. Mutation in the spectrin gene
D. Mutation in the protein 4.1 gene

Answer: A. A mutation in the lamin B receptor on chromosome 1 underlines the pathogenesis of familial Pelger–Huet anomaly. Mutations in the concanavalin-A receptor are implicated in Shwachman–Diamond syndrome. Spectrin abnormalities are part of the defect in hereditary spherocytosis and elliptocytosis, and protein 4.1 is similarly related to hereditary elliptocytosis.

CASE 95

A 28-year-old male presents with a 2-month history of fatigue and weakness. Physical exam reveals splenomegaly. Laboratory workup shows a leukocyte count of 274,000/μL, hemoglobin of 7.2g/dL, and a platelet count of 13,000/μL. A chest film is normal. The peripheral blood smear is shown. Flow cytometry shows expression of CD2+, CD3+, CD5+, CD7+, HLA-DR+, and TdT+. The peripheral blood smear is shown.

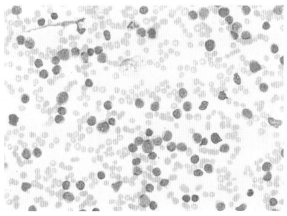
CASE FIGURE 95-1

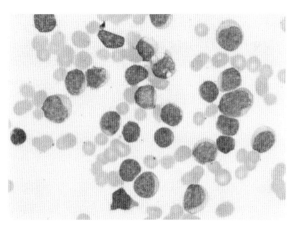
CASE FIGURE 95-2

QUESTION 1

☆ What is the most likely diagnosis?

A. B-cell acute lymphoblastic leukemia (B-ALL)
B. T-cell acute lymphoblastic leukemia (T-ALL)
C. Chronic myelogenous leukemia (CML)
D. Acute myeloid leukemia (AML)

Answer: B. The peripheral blood shows cells of variable size with a high nuclear–cytoplasmic ratio, indistinct nucleoli, fine to condensed chromatin, and round to irregular nuclei. The leukocyte morphology and immunophenotype are characteristic of T-ALL, which accounts for approximately 15% to 25% of adult ALL cases. Patients with T-ALL are older than patients with B-ALL and usually present with very high leukocyte counts, splenomegaly, and lymphadenopathy. A mediastinal mass maybe present. Adults with T-ALL may have a better prognosis than cases of B-ALL. B-ALL is usually positive for CD10, CD19, CD22, CD79a, HLA-DR, and TdT. The immunophenotype of AML is CD13+, CD33+, HLA-DR+, and CD34+. However, myeloid antigens may be expressed on lymphoblasts, and CD13 and CD33 have been described in ALL with the ETV6-RUNX1 mutation. The blood smear is not compatible with CML; there is no myeloid lift shift or basophilia.

QUESTION 2

☆ What molecular mutation is associated with the worst event-free survival in T-cell ALL?

A. NOTCH1
B. HOX11L.2
C. BCR-ABL
D. HOX11

Answer: B. HOX11L.2 confers a poor prognosis, with an event-free survival of 20% at 2 years. On the other hand, HOX11 is associated with a favorable outcome, with an estimated 70% to 80% disease-free survival at 3 years. Activating NOTCH1 mutations have been reported in more than 50% of T-ALL cases. They have not been associated with an unfavorable prognosis, and in fact some series have reported that this mutation may confer a good prognosis. BCR-ABL is observed in approximately 25% of adults with B-ALL and is an adverse prognostic factor.

Hemolysis, 30, 139
    cold agglutinin-induced, 103–104
    oxidative, cause of, 149
Hemolytic anemia, 73, 140
    with PK deficiency-associated, 111–112
    spur cell anemia as, 41–42
Hemolytic uremic syndrome (HUS), 196–197
Hemophagocytic lymphohistiocytosis (HLH)
        syndrome, 108, 132
Hemophagocytic syndrome, 20
Hemoptysis, 7
Hepatitis C, association with splenic marginal zone
        lymphoma, 86
Hepatoplenomegaly, 94
Hereditary elliptocytosis (HE), 12–13, 194
    defect in, 195
    hereditary spherocytosis, difference between, 195
Hereditary spherocytosis (HS), 18, 20
    hereditary elliptocytosis, difference between, 195
    molecular defect in, 19
    test to confirm, 19
High-dose cytarabine consolidation, 11
Histoplasmosis capsulatum, 66
HIV infection
    associated thrombotic thrombocytopenic purpura, 35
    disseminated histoplasmosis with, 65–66
    mycobacterium avium complex, 67–68
HLA-DR, 22
HLD-DR+, 9
HLH. *See* Hemophagocytic lymphohistiocytosis
HME. *See* Human monocytic erhlichiosis
Homocysteine, 13
Horse ATG (h-ATG), 75
Howell–Jolly bodies, 56–57, 146, 177
HOX11L.2 mutations, 208
Human granulocytic anaplasmosis (HGA), 156
    vs. human monocytic erhlichiosis, 156
    treatment for, 156
Human monocytic ehrlichiosis (HME), 155
    vs. human granulocytic anaplasmosis, 156
    treatment for, 156
Hydroxyurea
    adverse effects of, 148
    for essential thrombocytosis, 33
    sickle-beta(+) thalassemia, 148
Hypersplenism, 102, 177
    presence of, 187
Hyposegmented neutrophils, 177

I

IgG antibodies, 25, 204
IgM antibodies, 24, 25, 96, 104
ILCL. *See* Intravascular large cell lymphoma
Imatinib, 90, 173

Immune-mediated platelet destruction, 188
Immune thrombocytopenia (IT), 146, 160
    test for, 145
    treatments, 146
Immune thrombocytopenic purpura (ITP)
    and autoimmune hemolytic anemia, 105
        management of, 106
Immunophenotype
    of acute myeloid leukemia, 208
    Sezary syndrome, 201
Immunosuppressive agents, for large granular lymphocyte
        leukemia, 152
Ineffective erythropoiesis, 91
Infectious mononucleosis, 104
Interferon alfa, 88, 92
International Staging System (ISS), 142
Intravascular large cell lymphoma (ILCL), 136
Intravenous gamma globulins (IVIG), 73
Inv(16), 175
    acute myeloid leukemia with, 175–176
Iron-deficiency anemia, 32, 191
    microcytic, 6–7
Isochromosome 12p, 200
Isochromosome 17q, 173
ISS. *See* International Staging System
IVIG. *See* Intravenous gamma globulins

J

JAK2 mutation, 100, 173
    testing for, 32, 37, 100

K

KIT D816V mutation, 11, 64
    in acute myeloid leukemia, 11

L

Lamin B receptor, mutation in, 206
Large granular lymphocyte leukemia (LGL), 119, 151
    clinical presentation of, 151
    first- or second-line therapy in, 152
Lenalidomide, 70–71
Leukoerythroblastosis, 67, 83–84
Levamisole, 165
LGL. *See* Large granular lymphocyte leukemia
Loa loa, 189
Loiasis, 189–190
    coinfection, 190
Loxosceles reclusa, 114
Loxoscelism, 113–114
    hematologic manifestations of, 114
    treatment, 114
LPL. *See* Lymphoplasmacytic lymphoma